What If It's Not What You Think?

Rethinking Breast Health and Cancer Risks

MJ Revz

Copyright Statement

Disclaimer

The information provided in this eBook is intended for educational and informational purposes only and should not be considered medical advice. While every effort has been made to ensure the accuracy and reliability of the content, it is important to understand that individual health situations vary greatly. Always consult with a qualified healthcare professional before making any decisions regarding your health, treatment options, or lifestyle changes. The authors and publishers of this eBook do not assume any responsibility for any adverse effects or consequences resulting from the use or application of the information contained herein.

This eBook may include references to third-party sources and studies; however, the inclusion of such references does not imply endorsement or guarantee of accuracy. Readers are encouraged to seek further information and clarification from their healthcare providers regarding any concerns they may have. Your health is a personal journey, and the information provided here is meant to empower you to make informed choices in collaboration with your medical team. Thank you for taking the time to read this eBook, and we wish you well on your health journey.

Contents

Introduction 1

Worried About a Lump? Learn How to Evaluate Its Risk for Cancer. 6

Want to Take Charge of Your Breast Health? Learn the Secrets of an Effective Self-Exam 13

What are the Benefits of Regular Screening, and How is it Performed? 20

Family History Matters: Discover Your Hereditary Breast Cancer Risks 29

A Woman's Guide to Lymphadenectomy and Mastectomy...34

Facing a Breast Biopsy? Uncover the Steps, Types, and What to Expect! 43

Your Essential Guide to Understanding Breast Cancer Stages and Treatment Paths 63

Is Breast Cancer Curable? What Percentage of Cases Are Considered Curable? 69

Is There Hope for Recovery in Stage 4 Breast Cancer, and Can It Still Be Treated? 73

Thinking About the Costs of Breast Cancer Surgery? Here's the Ideal Estimation Cost You Should Know...82

Effective Strategies for Utilizing the Latest Technology in Breast Cancer Detection...............88

What Makes Histopathology Essential for Diagnosing Diseases? 95

What Resources Are Available for Individuals with Breast Cancer Who Cannot Afford Treatment, and How Can Loved Ones Help? 102

What foods should be avoided when you have breast cancer? 107

How many years must pass for someone to be considered cancer-free? 114

Is There a Possibility That Breast Cancer Will Return After Treatment Has Been Completed?..120

Is There Evidence Linking Underwire Bras or Antiperspirants to Increased Breast Cancer Risk? 125

Can Soursop, Mangosteen, and Green Tea Unlock the Secrets to Beating Breast Cancer? 127

Can Hormonal Therapy Cause Ovarian Thickening? Understanding Tamoxifen's Effects131

What Body Parts Should Be Monitored After Breast Cancer Treatment? 135

Your Guide to Pregnancy After Breast Cancer: Empowering Choices for the Future 140

Is Pain After Surgery and Tumor Removal a Side Effect? Understanding the Causes 146

Embracing Your Journey...................................150

Introduction

Imagine waking up one day, going about your usual routine, when you suddenly feel something unusual in your breast—a lump that wasn't there before. In that moment, a wave of emotions hits you: fear, confusion, and a million questions racing through your mind. Is it cancer? What does this mean for my life? This moment can mark the beginning of a journey that many women face—a journey filled with uncertainty but also with hope, strength, and the power to take charge of their health.

Globally, breast cancer is the most common cancer among women, with approximately **2.3 million new cases diagnosed in 2022 and around 670,000 deaths attributed to the disease that same year.** The lifetime risk of being diagnosed varies significantly by region; in high Human Development Index (HDI) countries, 1 in 12 women will be diagnosed, while in low HDI countries, the figure is 1 in 27. In 2024 alone, an estimated **310,720 women will be diagnosed with invasive breast cancer in the United States.** Understanding this disease is more crucial than ever as awareness and early detection can significantly improve survival rates.

This eBook is here to be your companion on this journey. Whether you're newly diagnosed, a survivor, or simply someone looking to learn more, you'll find valuable insights and practical information that can help guide you through this challenging time. The journey begins with awareness—recognizing what changes are happening in your body and knowing how to respond. Learning how to perform a self-exam is an empowering step. It's not just about finding lumps; it's about getting to know your body better and being proactive about your health. Regular screenings are also crucial; they can lead to early detection, which significantly improves treatment success rates.

As we dive deeper into this topic, we'll explore how family history can impact your risk for breast cancer. Understanding your family's medical background can provide important clues about your own health risks. Knowledge is power, and being aware of these factors can help you make informed decisions about your health moving forward. If you find yourself facing a breast cancer diagnosis, it can feel overwhelming. You might have questions swirling around in your head: What are my treatment options? What will surgery involve? In this eBook, we'll discuss various surgical choices—like lymphadenectomy versus mastectomy—

helping you weigh the pros and cons based on your unique situation.

We'll also tackle the financial aspects of breast cancer surgery, which can add stress to an already tough situation. When it's time for a biopsy, anxiety may set in. What should you expect? We'll guide you through the different types of biopsies available so that you can approach this step with confidence. Once diagnosed, understanding how breast cancer is staged becomes critical. Staging helps determine treatment plans and gives insight into what to expect moving forward. We'll break down the stages of breast cancer and what they mean for your treatment options.

One of the most pressing questions many have is whether breast cancer is curable. We'll explore survival rates based on stage and discuss what hope looks like at every step of this journey. Even if faced with advanced stages of cancer, there are treatment options available that can improve quality of life and extend survival. For those considering breast preservation options, we'll provide insights into when these choices are viable based on staging and tumor characteristics. Your body is unique, and understanding how to navigate these choices is essential for both physical and emotional well-being. Throughout this journey, support systems are invaluable. Recognizing that financial barriers can impact treatment decisions, we'll outline various resources available for individuals who cannot afford treatment—from government programs to charitable organizations. Emotional support from loved ones during this challenging time cannot be overstated; it often serves as the foundation upon which healing begins.

As you progress through treatment and recovery, nutrition becomes increasingly important. We'll discuss foods to avoid during treatment as well as those that can help boost your immune system—empowering you to take control of what you eat during this time. Emerging from treatment brings its own set of questions and challenges. Concerns about recurrence may linger long after treatment has ended. We'll address these concerns by discussing long-term monitoring and what signs to watch for after treatment. Additionally, we'll explore personal aspects of life after a diagnosis—such as intimacy and relationships—as well as the physical changes that may occur due to hormonal therapies or surgeries.

Throughout this eBook, we aim to debunk common myths surrounding breast cancer—like whether underwire bras or antiperspirants increase risk—and clarify misconceptions about natural remedies like soursop or green tea as cures for cancer. Finally, we will address practical concerns such as pain management after surgery and how hormonal therapy may affect ovarian health. This eBook isn't just a collection of facts; it's a roadmap designed to guide you through one of life's most challenging journeys with knowledge and empowerment at every turn. As you read through these pages, remember that you are not alone—there's a community ready to support you every step of the way. Let this eBook serve as both a resource and a source of inspiration as you navigate your path through breast cancer awareness, treatment options, recovery strategies, and beyond. Embrace each moment with hope and resilience; your story matters, and your journey is just beginning.

Worried About a Lump? Learn How to Evaluate Its Risk for Cancer.

Discovering a lump in your breast can be frightening, often leading to a whirlwind of emotions and questions. It's essential to remember that not all lumps are cancerous; many are benign. Knowing how to respond is crucial for your peace of mind and health.

Immediate Steps to Take After Discovering a Lump

- If you notice a lump, stay calm and assess it by asking yourself:
- Is it new?
- Has its size or shape changed?
- Does it feel different from the surrounding tissue?

These observations can provide valuable information when you consult a healthcare professional. Schedule an appointment with your doctor as soon as possible. Early detection is key in managing breast health. During your visit, your doctor will likely perform a physical examination and may recommend imaging tests, such as a mammogram or ultrasound, to clarify what's happening.

Understanding the Standard Evaluation Procedures

The standard procedure for evaluating a breast lump typically involves several steps:

1. **Initial Evaluation:** A clinical breast exam is performed by your healthcare provider.
2. **Imaging Tests:** A mammogram and breast ultrasound help determine if the lump is benign or suspicious.

3. **Biopsy:** If imaging results are inconclusive, a biopsy (core needle or surgical) is performed to obtain tissue for examination.

Treatment Options for Malignant and Benign Lumps

If a breast lump is confirmed as malignant (cancerous), treatment usually focuses on removing the tumor and preventing its spread:

Surgery: This may involve:

- **Lumpectomy:** Removing the tumor and a small margin of surrounding tissue.

- **Mastectomy:** Removing the entire breast if the cancer is extensive.

Additional Treatments: Post-surgery, treatments such as radiation therapy, chemotherapy, or hormonal therapy may be recommended to eliminate any remaining cancer cells.

In contrast, if a breast lump is benign (non-cancerous):

- **Monitoring:** No immediate treatment is usually necessary. Your doctor may recommend regular monitoring to check if the lump changes over time.

- **Surgery (if needed)**: If the benign lump causes discomfort or continues to grow, surgical removal might be considered.

Breast Cancer Treatment by Stage

Breast cancer treatment varies significantly depending on the stage of the disease. Here's an overview:

Stage 1 Breast Cancer

Characteristics: Tumor size up to 2 cm with no lymph node involvement.

Treatment Steps:

- Surgery (lumpectomy or mastectomy)
- Chemotherapy (4 to 6 cycles)
- Radiation Therapy (20 to 30 sessions)
- Hormonal Therapy (if hormone receptor-positive)

Estimated Costs

Overall Cost: Approximately $60,637 in the first year. Costs can vary significantly based on location and insurance coverage.

Stage 2A and 2B Breast Cancer

Characteristics: Tumor size ranges from 2 to 5 cm, possibly with lymph node involvement.

Treatment Steps:

- Surgery combined with chemotherapy
- Chemotherapy (4 to 6 cycles)
- Radiation Therapy (25 to 30 sessions)

Estimated Costs

Overall Cost: Approximately $82,121 in the first year.

Stage 3 Breast Cancer

Characteristics: Larger tumors or extensive lymph node involvement.

Treatment Steps:

- Neoadjuvant Chemotherapy before surgery
- Adjuvant Therapy post-surgery (6 to 8 cycles)

Estimated Costs

Overall Cost: Approximately $129,387 in the first year.

Stage 4 Breast Cancer

Characteristics: Cancer has spread to distant organs.

Treatment Steps:

- Systemic therapies including ongoing chemotherapy and targeted therapy

Estimated Costs

Overall Cost: Approximately $134,682 in the first year.

NOTE: *Costs can vary significantly based on location and insurance coverage.*

Key Considerations

Each treatment plan is personalized based on cancer characteristics and patient health. Early-stage treatments focus on curative intent, while advanced stages aim to manage symptoms and prolong life. Insurance coverage can significantly impact out-of-pocket expenses, so it's essential to consult with healthcare providers and insurance companies regarding financial responsibilities.

How to Determine If the Lump Might Be Cancerous

While waiting for your appointment, you may wonder whether the lump could be cancerous. Certain characteristics can help you assess its nature:

- Shape and Texture: Cancerous lumps are often hard, irregularly shaped, and may feel fixed compared to surrounding tissue. Benign lumps are usually smooth and movable.

- Size Changes: Monitor any changes in size over time; a lump that grows larger may warrant further investigation.

- Accompanying Symptoms: Look for changes in skin texture (like dimpling), discharge from the nipple (especially if bloody), or swelling nearby.

It's worth noting that approximately 80% of breast lumps are not cancerous; conditions like cysts or fibroadenomas are common and typically require minimal intervention. However, it's essential not to ignore any changes in your body.

When meeting with your healthcare provider, be prepared to discuss your findings openly. Share any relevant family history of breast cancer or other risk factors you may have. Your doctor may recommend further tests based on their findings during the examination.

Encouragement for Proactive Health Management

Finding a lump in your breast can be concerning, but taking immediate action is key. Stay calm, observe any changes, and consult with your healthcare provider promptly. By being proactive and informed about your health, you can navigate this challenging situation with greater confidence and clarity.

Have you noticed any changes in your breast health? Remember that **awareness is an important part of self-care!**

Want to Take Charge of Your Breast Health? Learn the Secrets of an Effective Self-Exam

Performing a breast self-exam (BSE) is not just a health check; it's an empowering ritual that allows you to connect with your body and take charge of your breast health. While it might seem intimidating at first, the process is straightforward and can be incredibly beneficial. This guide will walk you through the importance of self-exams, how to perform them effectively, and additional resources to support your breast health journey.

Why Self-Exams Matter

Breast self-exams are vital for early detection of changes in breast tissue. According to the American Cancer Society, about 1 in 8 women will be diagnosed with breast cancer in their lifetime. The good news? Early detection can significantly improve treatment outcomes. By regularly examining your breasts, you become more familiar with their normal state, making it easier to notice any changes that may arise.

Understanding Breast Health

Breast tissue consists of glandular tissue, fat, and connective tissue, leading to variations in size and texture. It's normal for breasts to have some lumps due to glandular tissue; however, any new lumps or changes should be reported to your healthcare provider. Knowing what's normal for you is key to identifying potential issues.

Finding the Right Time

Timing your self-exam can make a difference. The best time to perform a BSE is about a week after your menstrual period ends when your breasts are less likely to be swollen or tender. If you no longer have periods, choose a specific day each month—this helps turn the exam into a routine. Many women find it convenient to do their self-exam while showering or getting dressed.

Your Step-by-Step Guide

1. Start with Visual Inspection

Begin by standing in front of a mirror in a well-lit room. With your arms relaxed at your sides, take a moment to look at your breasts. Notice their shape and size—are they symmetrical? Look for any visible changes such as swelling, dimpling, or alterations in

skin texture. Next, raise your arms above your head
and observe again for any differences.

2. Feel Your Breasts While Lying Down

Now, lie down on your back. This position flattens the
breast tissue against the chest wall, making it easier to
feel for lumps or abnormalities. Use the pads of your
fingers—avoid using your fingertips—and start at the
outer edge of one breast. Move in circular motions
toward the nipple, applying different levels of
pressure:

- Light Pressure: For surface tissue.
- Medium Pressure: For deeper areas.
- Firm Pressure: For the chest wall beneath.

Make sure to cover the entire breast area
systematically.

3. Check While Standing or Sitting

You can also perform this exam while standing or
sitting if that feels more comfortable for you. Use the
same circular motions and varying pressure as when
lying down.

4. Don't Forget Your Armpits

Breast tissue extends into your armpits, so make sure to check this area as well. Feel for any lumps or unusual changes here.

Know What's Normal vs. Abnormal

Understanding what's normal versus abnormal in breast tissue is essential for effective self-exams. Each woman's breasts have unique characteristics; being familiar with your own anatomy allows you to notice any changes over time.

What's Normal?

Normal breast tissue can vary widely in texture and appearance. Many women may notice that their breasts feel lumpy or have areas of firmness due to glandular tissue, especially around their menstrual cycle. These variations are typically benign and part of normal breast structure. Additionally, it's common for one breast to be slightly larger than the other; this asymmetry is normal for most women.

What's Abnormal?

Abnormal changes may include new lumps, persistent changes in size or shape, or alterations in skin texture. For instance:

- **New Lump:** If you find a lump that wasn't there before and it feels different from surrounding tissue (such as being hard or fixed), it should be evaluated by a doctor.

- **Skin Changes:** If the skin on your breast develops a texture resembling an orange peel (known as peau d'orange) or shows signs of redness or swelling, these changes could indicate an underlying issue.

- **Nipple Changes:** Unusual discharge from your nipple (e.g., blood or clear fluid when it wasn't present before) is another reason to seek medical advice.

Common Concerns Addressed

What If I Find a Lump? If you notice something that feels different or persistent changes in size or shape, don't hesitate to reach out for medical advice.

Myths vs. Facts: Many women worry that self-exams are unnecessary if they have regular mammograms; however, BSEs complement clinical exams and help you stay attuned to your body.

Making Self-Exams Part of Your Routine

Incorporating breast self-exams into your monthly routine not only helps you stay informed about your body but also fosters empowerment and connection with yourself. Consider creating a simple log or using an app to track your self-exams and any changes you notice over time.

Encourage Regular Healthcare Visits

Remember that BSEs should complement regular clinical exams and mammograms—not replace them. Discussing your self-exam findings with your healthcare provider during routine check-ups can enhance overall breast health awareness.

Understanding Common Types of Breast Lumps

When it comes to breast lumps, understanding the different types and their behaviors is crucial for anyone concerned about their breast health:

- **Fibroadenomas:** Benign tumors typically appearing in young women (ages 15–35). They are firm, smooth, rubbery lumps that usually don't pose cancer risks.

- **Breast Cysts:** Fluid-filled sacs more common in women aged 35–60. These may fluctuate in size with hormonal changes but are also non-cancerous.

- **Atypical Hyperplasia:** A condition where abnormal cells grow in breast ducts or lobules; while not cancerous, it can increase future cancer risk.
- **Phyllodes Tumors:** Can be benign or malignant and often present as fast-growing lumps; they vary significantly in behavior.

While most breast lumps are benign, any new lump should be evaluated by a healthcare professional to rule out cancer. Breast cancer often presents as a firm lump that may not be painful and can occur at any age. Symptoms like changes in shape or skin texture, nipple discharge, or persistent pain should prompt immediate medical attention.

By being aware of these different types of lumps and their characteristics, individuals can take proactive steps toward their breast health and seek timely medical advice when necessary.

What are the Benefits of Regular Screening, and How is it Performed?

Regular screening for breast cancer is vital for maintaining breast health and can significantly impact outcomes. Many women wonder about the benefits of screening and how it works.

Benefits of Regular Screening

1. Early Detection: One of the most significant benefits is detecting breast cancer at an early stage when it is smaller and has not spread, making it easier to treat successfully. Early detection can lead to better treatment options and improved survival rates.

2. Increased Treatment Options: Early detection often provides more treatment options. Women diagnosed with early-stage breast cancer may be eligible for breast-conserving surgery (lumpectomy) instead of a mastectomy.

3. Reduced Mortality Rates: Studies show that regular screening can lower the risk of dying from breast cancer. Catching the disease early allows timely treatment that prevents cancer from advancing.

4. Peace of Mind: Regular screenings provide reassurance; knowing you are actively monitoring your health can alleviate anxiety about potential issues.

5. Monitoring Changes Over Time: Regular screenings enable healthcare providers to monitor changes in breast tissue over time, helping identify concerning developments early on, even if they don't yet show symptoms.

How Is Breast Cancer Screening Performed?

Breast cancer screening typically involves several methods, with mammography being the most common:

I. Mammography

A mammogram is an X-ray image used primarily to detect breast cancer early when it is most treatable. This method can identify tumors that are too small to be felt and reveal other abnormalities in breast tissue.

Two Main Types of Mammograms:

1. **Screening Mammograms:** Routine checks for women without symptoms, involving two X-ray images taken from different angles.

2. **Diagnostic Mammograms:** More detailed images used when symptoms such as a lump or unusual changes are present.

Why Are Mammograms Important?

The significance of mammograms cannot be overstated:

Early Detection Saves Lives: According to the American Cancer Society, regular mammograms can reduce breast cancer mortality by 20-30% among women aged 40 and older.

Localized Breast Cancer Survival Rate: The five-year survival rate for localized breast cancer (cancer that has not spread beyond the breast) is approximately 99%, underscoring the importance of regular screenings.

Understanding Your Risk

Breast cancer risk increases with age, particularly after 50. Other factors include family history, genetic predispositions (like BRCA1 and BRCA2 mutations), and lifestyle choices. Knowing your risk helps you make informed decisions about when to start screening.

American Cancer Society Recommendations

The American Cancer Society provides clear guidelines for mammogram screenings:

- Ages 40-44: Women should have the option to start annual screenings if they choose.

- Ages 45-54: Annual mammograms are recommended.

- Ages 55 and Older: Women can switch to biennial screenings or continue annual screenings based on personal preference.

These recommendations emphasize personalized healthcare decisions; discussing individual risk factors with your healthcare provider is essential.

Preparing for Your Mammogram

Proper preparation can ease anxiety about your mammogram:

- **Schedule Wisely:** Try to schedule your appointment when your breasts are less likely to be tender—typically one week after your menstrual period.

- **Avoid Certain Products:** Refrain from using deodorants, antiperspirants, lotions, or powders on your breasts or underarms before the exam, as these can interfere with X-ray images.

- **Wear Comfortable Clothing:** Opt for a two-piece outfit so you can easily undress from the waist up without discomfort.

What Happens During a Mammogram?

Understanding what occurs during a mammogram can help alleviate fears:

Check-In: Upon arrival at the imaging center, you will check in and complete necessary paperwork.

Changing Clothes: You'll change into a gown that opens in the front.

The Procedure:

You will stand in front of an X-ray machine.

A technologist will position your breast on a flat surface and compress it with a paddle—this compression lasts only a few seconds but is crucial for clear images.

Two images will be taken of each breast from different angles.

Duration: The entire process typically takes about 20 minutes.

Addressing Common Concerns

Many women worry about discomfort during the procedure; while some pressure is applied during compression, it usually lasts only briefly. Communicating any discomfort to the technologist can help adjust their technique.

After Your Mammogram

Once your mammogram is complete, results typically take a few days:

Normal Results: If no abnormalities are found, you will usually receive notification within a week.

Further Evaluation: If something suspicious is detected, your healthcare provider may recommend additional imaging or tests.

Understanding Your Results

Not all abnormalities indicate cancer; many may be benign conditions. However, follow-up testing is crucial for peace of mind and health management.

Overcoming Barriers to Screening

Despite its importance, many women do not get regular mammograms due to various barriers:

- **Fear and Anxiety:** Many fears potential pain or bad news; education about what to expect can alleviate these fears.

- **Cost and Access:** Some face financial barriers or lack access to facilities; programs exist offering free or low-cost screenings for eligible individuals.

- **Cultural Beliefs:** Cultural attitudes towards health screenings can also play a role; community outreach can help address these issues.

Empowering Yourself Through Knowledge

Knowledge is power when it comes to health decisions. By understanding what a mammogram entails and its importance in detecting breast cancer early, you empower yourself and those around you by encouraging friends and family members to prioritize their health through regular screenings.

II. Clinical Breast Exam (CBE)

A Clinical Breast Exam (CBE) is a physical examination performed by a trained healthcare provider to assess breasts for abnormalities such as lumps or changes in texture:

- **Visual Inspection:** You will sit or stand while the provider visually inspects your breasts for noticeable changes in size, shape, or skin texture.

- **Physical Examination:** The provider will feel your breasts while you lie down; this position helps flatten breast tissue for thorough examination using firm pressure to check for lumps or areas of thickening.

- **Assessment of Findings:** If any abnormalities are detected, the provider will discuss findings with you and may recommend follow-up tests.

- **Frequency Recommendations:** The American Cancer Society does not recommend routine CBEs for average-risk women at any age but suggests that women in their 20s and 30s have a CBE every one to three years during regular check-ups while women aged 40 and older should prioritize annual mammograms instead.

Importance of Clinical Breast Exams

While mammograms are primary screening tools recommended for detecting breast cancer in average-risk women, CBEs still play a role in overall breast health management:

- **Complementary Role:** CBEs can help identify changes not visible on imaging tests; they are particularly important if unusual changes occur between screenings.
- **Education and Awareness:** A CBE provides an opportunity for healthcare providers to educate patients about breast health and self-examination techniques, empowering them to recognize potential issues early.

In summary, while Clinical Breast Exams are important for breast health care, they should not replace regular mammograms as a screening method for average-risk women. Consult with your healthcare provider regarding appropriate frequency tailored to your needs if you have concerns about your breast health or specific risk factors.

Family History Matters: Discover Your Hereditary Breast Cancer Risks

Have you ever wondered if your family history might indicate a risk for breast cancer? Understanding hereditary factors is essential for many women, particularly regarding genetic mutations like BRCA1 and BRCA2, which significantly influence breast cancer risk.

What Are BRCA1 and BRCA2?

BRCA1 and BRCA2 are crucial genes found in everyone's DNA. Their primary role is to produce proteins that repair damaged DNA in our cells. Think of these genes as the body's "repair crew" for genetic material. When functioning correctly, they help keep our cells healthy and prevent uncontrolled growth that can lead to cancer.

How Do They Work?

To visualize how BRCA1 and BRCA2 function, imagine your DNA as blueprints for constructing a building. Just as builders must fix mistakes in blueprints to ensure safety and stability, BRCA proteins correct errors in our DNA to prevent problems.

When these genes work properly, they act like safety nets that catch mistakes before they escalate into serious issues. However, if a mutation occurs—altering the gene's function—the repair crew can't perform effectively, leading to an increased risk of cancers, particularly breast and ovarian cancers.

What Happens When There's a Mutation?

Mutations in the BRCA1 or BRCA2 genes can significantly raise breast cancer risk:

- **Women with a BRCA1 mutation** have about a 55-65% chance of developing breast cancer by age 70.

- **Women with a BRCA2 mutation** face about a 45% chance.

- In contrast, the general population has only a 12% chance of developing breast cancer in their lifetime.

For example, if part of your house's foundation is cracked (the mutation) and remains unfixed (the repair process), the entire structure could become unstable over time (leading to cancer).

Why Is This Important?

Understanding BRCA1 and BRCA2 is crucial because these mutations can be passed down from parents to children. If someone inherits a mutated version from a parent, every cell in their body will have one normal copy and one mutated copy. If both copies fail, this significantly increases cancer risk.

For instance, if your mother has a BRCA1 mutation, you have about a 50% chance of inheriting that mutation yourself. This highlights the importance of considering genetic testing if there's a family history of breast or ovarian cancer.

Who Should Consider Genetic Testing?

Genetic testing is advisable for women with:

- A family history of breast or ovarian cancer.

- Multiple relatives on one side affected by these cancers.

- A personal history of breast cancer diagnosed before age 50.

- Close relatives (mother or sister) who had breast cancer at an early age.

If you meet any of these criteria, discussing genetic testing with your healthcare provider is essential.

Genetic counseling can also provide valuable insights into the implications of testing.

Making Informed Health Decisions

Testing positive for a BRCA mutation can lead to challenging health management decisions. Options include:

- **Increased Surveillance:** More frequent mammograms or MRIs to monitor for signs of cancer.

- **Preventive Surgeries:** Procedures such as mastectomy (removal of breasts) or oophorectomy (removal of ovaries) to reduce cancer risk.

Open discussions with healthcare professionals can help tailor strategies to individual situations. Knowledge about hereditary risks empowers women to make informed choices about their health.

The Importance of Family History

While most breast cancer cases are not hereditary, understanding your family history is vital. Women with first-degree relatives (mother or sister) who have had breast cancer nearly double their risk; the more relatives affected, the higher the risk becomes.

Additionally, men can also carry BRCA mutations and have an increased risk for breast cancer and other cancers such as prostate and pancreatic cancer.

Understanding hereditary factors like BRCA1 and BRCA2 mutations can significantly impact your health decisions. If you have concerns about your family history or genetic risks for breast cancer, consult your healthcare provider for advice and potential testing options. Being proactive about your health can lead to better outcomes and peace of mind.

A Woman's Guide to Lymphadenectomy and Mastectomy

Breast cancer presents a complex journey for many women, often filled with questions and uncertainties. Among the most critical decisions are those regarding surgical options like lymphadenectomy and mastectomy. This guide aims to provide clear, informative insights into these procedures, empowering women to make informed choices about their health.

What You Need to Know

Mastectomy is the surgical removal of one or both breasts, usually to treat breast cancer. There are several types of mastectomy:

1. **Total (or Simple) Mastectomy:** Removal of the entire breast without lymph node involvement.

2. **Modified Radical Mastectomy:** Removal of the entire breast along with some lymph nodes under the arm.

3. **Radical Mastectomy:** An extensive procedure that removes the entire breast, lymph nodes, and chest wall muscles; this is

less common today due to advancements in treatment.

Lymphadenectomy is the surgical removal of lymph nodes to assess whether cancer has spread beyond the breast. This procedure is often performed alongside mastectomy or lumpectomy when there's concern about metastasis.

Why Are These Surgeries Essential?

Both procedures aim to effectively treat breast cancer. A mastectomy may be recommended for several reasons:

- Tumor Characteristics: Large tumors or multiple tumors in one breast may necessitate a mastectomy for effective removal.

- Personal Choice: Some women opt for mastectomy to alleviate anxiety about cancer recurrence.

- Genetic Considerations: Women with BRCA1 or BRCA2 mutations may choose preventive (prophylactic) mastectomies to reduce their risk.

Lymphadenectomy helps determine cancer staging by assessing nearby lymph nodes, providing vital information for future treatment planning.

Ideal Tumor Size for Mastectomy and Lymphadenectomy

Mastectomy is generally indicated for larger tumors or those with specific characteristics that make breast-conserving surgery less viable:

- T1: Tumors less than 2 cm (approximately 0.8 inches) may be candidates for breast-conserving surgery if no other contraindications exist.

- T2: Tumors between 2 cm and 5 cm (about 0.8 to 2 inches) can also be considered for lumpectomy depending on individual circumstances.

- T3: Tumors larger than 5 cm (approximately 2 inches) typically indicate a higher stage of cancer and are more likely to necessitate a mastectomy.

- T4: Any tumor that has invaded surrounding structures is classified as T4 and usually requires mastectomy due to its advanced nature.

Specific indications for mastectomy include tumors greater than 5 cm (T3) or multicentric disease where multiple tumors exist in the same breast.

Lymphadenectomy Considerations

Lymphadenectomy is typically performed when there is concern about cancer spread to nearby lymph nodes. For patients undergoing mastectomy with tumors larger than 5 cm or those with positive lymph nodes, lymphadenectomy is usually indicated to assess the extent of cancer spread.

Summary of Recommendations

1. For Tumors Less Than 2 cm (T1): Breast-conserving surgery may be an option if clear margins can be achieved.

2. For Tumors Between 2 cm and 5 cm (T2): Lumpectomy may still be considered depending on individual circumstances.

3. For Tumors Greater Than 5 cm (T3): Mastectomy is typically recommended due to increased risk of metastasis.

4. For T4 Tumors: Mastectomy is generally necessary due to local invasion.

Weighing Risks and Side Effects: What to Expect

Understanding potential risks and side effects associated with these surgeries is crucial. Common risks include:

- Infection: Risk of infection at the incision site.

- Bleeding: Some patients may experience excessive bleeding during or after surgery.

- Post-operative Pain: Most women experience some level of discomfort post-surgery.

A significant concern specific to lymphadenectomy is lymphedema, characterized by swelling due to fluid buildup when lymph nodes are removed. Preventive measures, such as avoiding heavy lifting and wearing compression garments if recommended, can help manage this risk.

Recovery Process

Recovery varies based on individual circumstances but generally includes:

- Hospital Stay: Most women stay in the hospital for 1-3 days post-surgery.

- Follow-Up Care: Regular follow-up appointments are essential for monitoring recovery and addressing complications.

- Gradual Return to Activity: Patients are encouraged to start gentle movements soon after surgery but should avoid strenuous activities for several weeks.

Women often seek guidance on managing pain and caring for surgical sites. Pain management strategies may include prescribed medications, ice packs, and a gradual return to normal activities as tolerated.

Future Treatments: How Surgery Influences Your Path Forward

Understanding how these surgeries will affect future treatments is a common concern. The presence of cancer in lymph nodes can significantly influence treatment decisions:

1. Chemotherapy: If cancer has spread to lymph nodes, oncologists may recommend chemotherapy to reduce recurrence risk.

2. Radiation Therapy: Women who undergo modified radical mastectomy may require radiation therapy targeting remaining cancer cells in the chest wall or underarm area.

Being informed about how these procedures fit into an overall treatment plan helps women feel more empowered in their healthcare decisions.

Addressing Psychological Impacts

The emotional impact of undergoing a mastectomy or lymphadenectomy can be profound. Many women experience feelings of loss related to body image and femininity. Common emotional responses include:

- Anxiety and Fear: Concerns about cancer recurrence can lead to heightened anxiety.

- Depression: Some women may experience depression following surgery due to physical changes or fear about their health.

- Body Image Issues: Physical changes resulting from surgery can affect self-esteem.

Support systems play a crucial role in helping women navigate these feelings. Many seek counseling or join support groups where they can share experiences with others who understand their journey. Engaging in open discussions with healthcare providers about emotional health is equally important.

Finding Support and Resources

Women facing decisions about lymphadenectomy and mastectomy should seek information from reliable sources. Organizations such as the American Cancer Society and Breastcancer.org offer valuable resources on understanding breast cancer treatments, coping strategies, and connecting with support groups. Additionally, discussing concerns with healthcare professionals—surgeons, oncologists, nurses—can provide personalized insights that empower women throughout their treatment journey.

Embracing Your Journey with Knowledge and Strength

Navigating a diagnosis of breast cancer is undoubtedly challenging. Understanding procedures like lymphadenectomy and mastectomy helps demystify treatment options and fosters informed decision-making. By addressing common concerns regarding risks, recovery, future treatments, and emotional impacts, women can better prepare themselves for what lies ahead. Ultimately, knowledge empowers women in their fight against breast cancer, enabling them to take control of their health journey with confidence.

Facing a Breast Biopsy? Uncover the Steps, Types, and What to Expect!

If you experience breast symptoms or if imaging tests, such as a mammogram, indicate potential breast cancer, your doctor may recommend a breast biopsy. This procedure involves removing small samples of breast tissue from the suspicious area for laboratory examination to determine the presence of cancer cells.

Understanding Breast Biopsies

A breast biopsy is a definitive method to diagnose breast conditions. Importantly, needing a biopsy does not automatically imply a cancer diagnosis; in fact, approximately 80% of biopsies yield benign results. However, a biopsy is the only reliable way to confirm or rule out breast cancer.

Types of Breast Biopsies

There are several types of breast biopsies, and the choice of procedure depends on various factors, including the characteristics of the suspicious area and patient preferences. The main types include:

1. Fine Needle Aspiration (FNA)

Fine Needle Aspiration (FNA) is a minimally invasive procedure used to assess suspicious lumps in the breast. This technique involves using a very thin, hollow needle to extract a small sample of tissue or fluid from the area of concern. FNA is often employed when imaging tests suggest the presence of breast cancer, although it is typically considered when other methods, like core needle biopsies, may not be suitable.

What to Expect During an FNA

Preparation and Procedure:
Before the procedure, your healthcare provider will discuss the lump with you, including its location and any changes you've noticed. You'll have the opportunity to ask questions and express any concerns. The FNA is usually performed in an outpatient setting, often in your doctor's office.

- Numbing the Area: While local anesthesia may be used to numb the area, it's not always necessary due to the thinness of the needle.

- Positioning: You will lie on your back during the procedure. If ultrasound guidance is used, you may feel some pressure from the ultrasound wand as the needle is inserted.

- Sample Collection: The doctor will insert the needle into the lump and withdraw a small amount of tissue or fluid. This process may be repeated several times to ensure an adequate sample is collected. Each sample takes about 15 seconds, and the entire procedure typically lasts around 20 to 30 minutes.

After the FNA

Following the procedure, you may experience some soreness at the biopsy site. Your doctor will provide instructions on how to care for the area and may recommend limiting strenuous activities for a day or so. Common side effects include minor bruising or swelling, which usually resolve over time. If you notice any unusual symptoms like persistent swelling or fever, it's important to contact your healthcare provider.

Understanding FNA Results

The samples taken during an FNA are sent to a pathologist for analysis to determine if cancer cells are present. The main advantages of FNA include its quick execution and minimal invasiveness—there's no need for stitches or incisions, which means less scarring.

However, there are limitations:

- Sample Size: FNA only collects a small amount of tissue, which may not provide enough information for a definitive diagnosis.

- False Negatives: There's a small chance that cancer cells could be missed if they are not included in the sample.

If the results from an FNA are inconclusive or if further testing is required, your doctor may recommend additional procedures, such as a core needle biopsy or surgical biopsy.

2. Core Needle Biopsy

A Core Needle Biopsy (CNB) is a common procedure used to evaluate suspicious breast abnormalities, particularly when imaging tests suggest the possibility of breast cancer. This biopsy method is preferred because it removes more tissue than a Fine Needle Aspiration (FNA) while avoiding the need for surgical intervention.

What is a Core Needle Biopsy?

During a CNB, a doctor uses a hollow needle to extract small cylindrical samples of breast tissue from the area of concern. The needle may be guided by the doctor's physical examination or by imaging techniques such as mammography, ultrasound, or MRI. In some cases, the needle is attached to a spring-loaded device that rapidly moves in and out of the tissue, or it may use suction to help draw tissue into the needle.

What to Expect During the Procedure

- **Setting:** A CNB is typically performed as an outpatient procedure in a doctor's office or clinic.

- **Preparation:** Before starting, the doctor will administer a local anesthetic to numb the area. A small incision (about ¼ inch) may be made in the skin to facilitate needle insertion.

- **Biopsy Process:** You may be positioned lying flat or on your side, depending on the imaging method used. The doctor will insert the needle into the breast tissue and remove several samples. You might feel pressure during this process.

- Marker Placement: A tiny marker (clip) may be placed at the biopsy site to help locate it in future imaging studies.

Aftercare

Post-procedure, you can generally resume normal activities within a day, although strenuous activities should be limited initially. Common side effects include bruising and swelling around the biopsy site, which typically resolve over time. Your healthcare provider will give you specific care instructions and advise you on what symptoms to monitor.

Types of Image-Guided Core Needle Biopsies

- **Stereotactic Biopsy:** This method uses mammogram images taken from different angles to pinpoint the biopsy site, often for small masses or microcalcifications.

- **Ultrasound-Guided Biopsy:** This technique utilizes ultrasound imaging to visualize the area being biopsied, allowing for real-time guidance.

- **MRI-Guided Biopsy:** Used when abnormalities are detected on an MRI that may not be visible on other imaging tests.

What Does a CNB Show?

The tissue samples obtained during a CNB are examined by a pathologist for cancer cells. CNBs are generally effective at providing clear diagnoses; however, there is still a risk of missing some cancers if they are not adequately sampled. If results are inconclusive or if there are ongoing concerns, further testing such as an additional CNB or surgical biopsy may be necessary.

3. Surgical (Open) Biopsy:

A surgical breast biopsy is a procedure used to find out if a suspicious area in the breast has cancer. This method is often used when other tests, like core needle biopsies or fine needle aspirations, don't give clear answers.

What is a Surgical Breast Biopsy?

In a surgical breast biopsy, a doctor removes a larger piece of breast tissue through a small cut in the skin. There are two main types:

1. **Excisional Biopsy:** The doctor removes the entire lump and some surrounding healthy tissue. This helps ensure that if there is cancer, it is all taken out.

2. **Incisional Biopsy:** Only part of the lump is removed for testing.

How Does the Procedure Work?

If the lump can't be felt, doctors use imaging tests (like mammograms or ultrasounds) to help guide them. For example, they might use a thin wire to mark the spot before surgery. This wire helps the surgeon know exactly where to cut.

What Happens During the Procedure?

- **Anesthesia:** You'll receive medicine to numb the area so you don't feel pain.

- **Incision:** The doctor makes a small cut in your breast and removes the suspicious tissue.

- **Stitches:** After removing the tissue, the doctor may put in stitches to close the cut and cover it with a bandage.

The whole procedure usually takes about 30 minutes to an hour.

Recovery

After the biopsy, you might notice some swelling or bruising around the area, which is normal and should go away in a few days. Your doctor will give you instructions on how to take care of the area and when you can return to your regular activities.

Getting Results

The tissue sample is sent to a specialist called a pathologist, who looks for cancer cells under a microscope. It usually takes several days to get results.

Example: If your biopsy shows no cancer cells, your doctor will discuss any follow-up tests you might need. If cancer is found, they will talk about treatment options.

4. Lymph Node Biopsy

A lymph node biopsy, specifically a sentinel lymph node biopsy (SLNB), is a crucial procedure used to determine if breast cancer has spread to the lymph nodes in the underarm area (axillary lymph nodes). This biopsy helps stage the cancer and guides treatment decisions.

What is a Sentinel Lymph Node Biopsy?

The sentinel lymph nodes are the first nodes that cancer cells are likely to spread to from the breast. During an SLNB, a doctor removes one or more of these nodes to check for the presence of cancer.

How Does the Procedure Work?

Preparation: Before the procedure, a radioactive substance and/or blue dye is injected into the breast. This helps identify the sentinel lymph nodes during surgery.

Surgery: The surgeon makes a small incision in the underarm area to remove the identified sentinel nodes. If cancer is found in these nodes, additional lymph nodes may be removed.

Recovery: The procedure is usually done on an outpatient basis, meaning you can go home the same day. Most people can return to their normal activities within a few days.

Why Is It Important?

The results of an SLNB can significantly impact treatment options:

- **Negative Result:** If no cancer is found in the sentinel nodes, it's unlikely that cancer has spread to other lymph nodes, and further surgery may not be needed.

- **Positive Result:** If cancer is detected, your doctor may recommend removing more lymph nodes (axillary lymph node dissection) or other treatments like chemotherapy or radiation.

Example 1

Imagine a woman diagnosed with early-stage breast cancer. During her surgery to remove the tumor, her doctor performs an SLNB. After injecting **dye** and locating the sentinel nodes, they find that none of these nodes contain cancer. This result means she may avoid more invasive surgery and can focus on her recovery and other treatments.

Importance of Dye in Sentinel Lymph Node Biopsy

In a sentinel lymph node biopsy (SLNB), a dye plays a crucial role in identifying the sentinel lymph nodes, which are the first nodes to which cancer cells are likely to spread from a tumor. This procedure is vital for determining whether breast cancer has metastasized, guiding treatment options accordingly.

How the Dye Works

- **Injection:** Before the biopsy, a harmless dye (commonly methylene blue or isosulfan blue) is injected near the tumor site. This dye travels through the lymphatic system to the sentinel lymph nodes.

- **Identification:** The sentinel nodes absorb the dye and become visibly stained. During surgery, the surgeon can easily locate these nodes due to their distinct color, allowing for their removal and further examination.

Advantages of Using Dye

- **Accuracy:** The use of dye significantly enhances the accuracy of identifying sentinel lymph nodes. Studies show that using methylene blue alone can achieve an identification rate of about 91%, with a sensitivity of 87% for detecting cancerous cells4. This means that most sentinel nodes can be accurately located and assessed for cancer.

- **Cost-Effectiveness:** Methylene blue is relatively inexpensive and readily available, especially in developing countries. This makes it a practical choice for hospitals with limited resources.

- **Reduced Morbidity:** By accurately identifying sentinel nodes, unnecessary removal of additional lymph nodes can be avoided. This minimizes surgical complications and long-term side effects, such as lymphedema (swelling due to fluid buildup) that can occur after more extensive surgeries.

- **Real-Time Guidance:** The dye provides immediate visual feedback during surgery, allowing surgeons to make informed decisions on-the-spot about which nodes to remove.

Example 2

Imagine a woman diagnosed with breast cancer. Before her surgery, her doctor injects methylene blue dye around the tumor. During the operation, the surgeon sees that the sentinel lymph nodes are stained blue. By removing these specific nodes for testing, they can quickly determine if cancer has spread without needing to remove all nearby lymph nodes.

Questions to Ask Before a Breast Biopsy

1. What type of biopsy do you recommend, and why?

    - Understanding the specific type of biopsy helps you know what to expect and why it's the best option for your situation.

2. How will the size of my breast affect the biopsy procedure?

    - This question addresses any concerns regarding how breast size might influence the technique or outcome of the biopsy.

3. Where will the biopsy be performed?

    - Knowing the location (hospital, outpatient center, etc.) can help you prepare logistically for the procedure.

4. What exactly will happen during the biopsy?

    - This helps set expectations and alleviate anxiety by providing a clear picture of the procedure.

5. How much tissue will be removed during the biopsy?

- Understanding the extent of tissue removal can clarify potential impacts on your breast and recovery.

6. How long will the procedure take?

   - Knowing the duration helps you plan your day and manage any related commitments.

7. Will I be awake during the procedure?
   - This question addresses sedation options and what level of consciousness you will have during the biopsy.

8. Will the area being biopsied be numbed?

   - Understanding pain management measures is crucial for comfort during the procedure.

9. If the abnormal area cannot be felt, how will you locate it?

   - This informs you about imaging techniques (like ultrasound or mammogram) that will be used to guide the biopsy.

10. Will a guide wire be used, and how will its placement be confirmed?

- Knowing how precision is ensured can reduce anxiety about potential errors in locating the abnormality.

11. Do I need someone to accompany me home afterward?

- This is important for planning post-procedure logistics, especially if sedation is involved.

12. Will there be a visible hole or scar after the procedure?

- Understanding cosmetic outcomes can help manage expectations regarding physical changes.

13. How will my breast look after the biopsy? Will it change shape?

- This addresses concerns about aesthetic changes and helps you prepare mentally for post-procedure appearances.

14. Will a clip or marker be placed in my breast, and what happens to it afterward?

- Knowing about markers can clarify their purpose and whether they will require future attention.

15. Will there be scarring, and where will it be located? What will it look like?
- This question provides insight into potential long-term effects on your breast's appearance.

16. What kind of bruising or skin discoloration should I expect, and how long will it last?

- Understanding possible side effects can help you prepare for your recovery period.

17. How much pain or soreness should I anticipate, and for how long?

- This helps set realistic expectations for post-biopsy discomfort and pain management strategies.

18. What complications should I watch for after the biopsy that would require contacting your office?

- Being informed about potential issues enables prompt action if complications arise.

19. When can I remove the bandage after the procedure?

  - Knowing when to remove dressings aids in proper wound care and healing.

20. When can I shower or bathe after the biopsy?

  - This information is crucial for maintaining hygiene while ensuring proper healing.

21. Will I have stitches, and if so, will they dissolve or need removal?

  - Understanding stitch care is important for recovery management.

22. When can I return to work, and how might I feel when I do?
  - This helps you plan your return to normal activities based on expected recovery time.

23. Are there any activity restrictions post-biopsy, such as lifting or raising my arm? If so, for how long?

- Knowing limitations helps prevent complications during recovery.

24. How soon can I expect to receive biopsy results?
    - Setting expectations for result timelines reduces anxiety about waiting for critical information.

25. Who will contact me with my results—will it be you or someone else?

    - Clarifying communication channels ensures you know whom to expect updates from regarding your health status.

26. Will you explain my biopsy results to me personally or refer me to someone else for this discussion?

    - Understanding who will provide results helps ensure that you receive comprehensive information directly from a knowledgeable source.

These questions are designed to empower patients with knowledge about their procedure, alleviate anxiety, and ensure they are fully informed about their care process before undergoing a breast biopsy.

Your Essential Guide to Understanding Breast Cancer Stages and Treatment Paths

When someone is diagnosed with breast cancer, understanding the stage of the cancer is crucial for determining treatment options and prognosis. Staging helps assess how advanced the cancer is and involves several key factors:

- Size of the tumor

- Spread to nearby lymph nodes

- Metastasis to other parts of the body

Breast cancer is typically classified into five stages, from Stage 0 to Stage IV.

What Is Staging?

Staging is the process of determining how far cancer has spread in the body. The TNM system (Tumor, Node, Metastasis) is commonly used to classify breast cancer stages.

The Stages of Breast Cancer

1. Stage 0: Ductal Carcinoma in Situ (DCIS)

Description: Abnormal cells are present in the lining of a breast duct but have not invaded surrounding tissues. This stage is non-invasive and highly treatable.

Recommended Actions:
- Surgery: Lumpectomy or mastectomy.

- Radiation Therapy: Often recommended post-lumpectomy.

- Monitoring: Regular follow-ups and imaging.

2. Stage I

Description: The tumor is small (up to 2 cm) and has not spread outside the breast. There may be some involvement of nearby lymph nodes.

Recommended Actions:
- Surgery: Lumpectomy or mastectomy.

- Radiation Therapy: Typically, after lumpectomy.
- Hormonal Therapy: If hormone receptor-positive, consider treatments like tamoxifen.
- Follow-Up Care: Regular check-ups and mammograms.

3. Stage II

This stage is divided into two sub-stages:

1. Stage IIA: Tumor size between 2 and 5 cm or spread to 1-3 nearby lymph nodes.

2. Stage IIB: Tumor larger than 5 cm but not spread to lymph nodes.

Recommended Actions:
Surgery: Lumpectomy or mastectomy.
Chemotherapy/Radiation: Often follows surgery based on individual assessment.

4. Stage III

Indicates a more advanced form of breast cancer, divided into sub-stages:

Stage IIIA: Spread to 1-3 nearby lymph nodes; no distant spread.

Recommended Actions:
- Neoadjuvant Chemotherapy: To shrink tumors before surgery.
- Surgery: Lumpectomy or mastectomy.
- Radiation Therapy: Post-surgery to target remaining cells.
- Hormonal/Targeted Therapy: If applicable.

Stage IIIB

Cancer has spread to nearby tissues (like chest wall or skin).

Recommended Actions:
- Similar to Stage IIIA with an emphasis on mastectomy and radiation therapy.

Stage IIIC

Extensive lymph node involvement without distant metastasis.

<u>Recommended Actions:</u>

- Neoadjuvant chemotherapy followed by surgery and radiation.

Stage IV: Metastatic Breast Cancer

Description: Cancer has spread beyond the breast and nearby lymph nodes to other body parts (e.g., bones, liver, lungs).

<u>Recommended Actions:</u>

- Systemic Treatments: Focus on chemotherapy, targeted therapy, or hormone therapy for disease control.

- Palliative Care: Manage symptoms and improve quality of life.

- Clinical Trials: Consider participation for access to new treatments.

- Regular Follow-Up Care: Ongoing monitoring for treatment effectiveness.

Why Is Staging Important?

Understanding the stage of breast cancer is essential because it guides treatment decisions:

- Early-stage cancers (Stages 0-I) may be effectively treated with surgery alone.

- Locally advanced cancers (Stages II-III) often require a combination of treatments for better outcomes.

- Metastatic cancers (Stage IV) necessitate ongoing management strategies aimed at symptom control and prolonging life.

Emotional Support

It's also important for patients to seek emotional support throughout their journey. Counseling services, support groups, and mental health resources can provide valuable assistance in coping with diagnosis and treatment

Is Breast Cancer Curable? What Percentage of Cases Are Considered Curable?

When faced with a breast cancer diagnosis, many people wonder about the possibility of a cure. The good news is that breast cancer is highly treatable, especially when detected early. However, the likelihood of achieving a complete cure can vary based on several factors, including the stage of cancer at diagnosis and the specific type of breast cancer involved.

Understanding Remission

Before diving into curability, it's important to grasp the concept of remission. When doctors refer to a patient being in remission, they mean there has been a significant decrease or disappearance of cancer signs and symptoms. There are two main types of remission:

1. **Partial Remission:** The cancer has shrunk but is still present in some form.

2. **Complete Remission:** All signs of cancer have vanished, and tests show no detectable cancer cells.

While doctors may consider a patient cured if no signs of the disease are found after a certain period, they rarely guarantee that cancer will never return.

Survival Rates by Stage

The potential for curing breast cancer often hinges on its stage at diagnosis. Here's how different stages impact treatment outcomes:

- **Stage 1:** Characterized by localized cancerous cells that have invaded surrounding breast tissue but have not spread beyond the breast. Treatment typically involves surgery (lumpectomy or mastectomy), often followed by radiation therapy. In many cases, chemotherapy or hormonal therapy may also be recommended to reduce the risk of recurrence. Generally, Stage 1 breast cancer is considered highly curable, with survival rates around 99%.

- **Stage 2:** The tumor may be larger or have spread to nearby lymph nodes. Treatment usually combines surgery, chemotherapy, radiation therapy, and hormonal therapy. This stage is also regarded as curable with effective treatment options available, boasting survival rates of approximately 86%.

- **Stage 3:** Indicates more advanced disease where the tumor has spread to several lymph nodes and possibly nearby tissues. Treatment becomes more aggressive and may involve neoadjuvant chemotherapy (given before surgery) followed by surgery and radiation therapy afterward. While Stage 3 breast cancer is more challenging to treat than earlier stages, it can still be curable with appropriate interventions; survival rates are around 66-98%, depending on various factors.

- **Stage 4:** Represents metastatic breast cancer, where the disease has spread to other parts of the body such as bones, liver, or lungs. At this stage, while treatments can help manage symptoms and prolong life, they typically do not cure the disease. Instead, therapies focus on controlling the cancer as a chronic condition through systemic treatments like chemotherapy and targeted therapies. The survival rate for Stage 4 breast cancer is about 31%.

Survival Statistics Overview

Survival rates provide valuable insight into how well patients respond to treatment based on their specific stage at diagnosis:

Stage	Description	5-Year Survival Rate
Stage 1	Localized (not spread beyond the breast)	~99%
Stage 2	Spread to nearby lymph nodes	~86-90%
Stage 3	More extensive involvement with lymph nodes	~66-98%
Stage 4	Metastatic (spread to distant organs)	~31%

These statistics illustrate the importance of early detection and effective treatment options in improving outcomes for patients diagnosed with breast cancer.

Is There Hope for Recovery in Stage 4 Breast Cancer, and Can It Still Be Treated?

Receiving a diagnosis of stage 4 breast cancer can feel like a heavy weight on your shoulders. It's a moment that can shake you to your core, as this stage means the cancer has spread beyond the breast and nearby lymph nodes to other parts of the body, such as the bones, liver, lungs, or brain. But amidst the fear and uncertainty, it's important to remember that there is still hope and effective treatment options available.

What Does Stage 4 Breast Cancer Mean?

Stage 4 breast cancer signifies an advanced state of the disease. While it may not be curable in the traditional sense, many people continue to live long, meaningful lives with proper management. The focus shifts from trying to eliminate the disease completely to controlling it and enhancing quality of life. According to the American Cancer Society, the 5-year relative survival rate for stage 4 breast cancer is about 31%. This statistic reminds us that while this stage is serious, many patients can manage their condition effectively.

Factors That Affect Prognosis

Understanding your prognosis can be empowering. Several factors can influence how well someone responds to treatment:

- Hormone Receptor Status: Cancers that are hormone receptor-positive (HR+) often respond better to hormonal therapies.

- HER2 Status: HER2-positive cancers may respond well to targeted therapies like trastuzumab (Herceptin).

- Overall, Health: A patient's general health and age can significantly impact treatment options and outcomes.

- Response to Treatment: How well a patient responds to initial treatments can guide future therapy decisions.

By discussing these factors with your healthcare team, you can gain insight into what might work best for you.

Exploring Treatment Options

When it comes to treating stage 4 breast cancer, there are several systemic therapies available. These treatments work throughout the body to target cancer cells and include chemotherapy, hormonal therapy, targeted therapy, immunotherapy, radiation therapy, and sometimes surgery.

1. Chemotherapy

Chemotherapy involves powerful medications designed to kill fast-growing cancer cells.

How It Works: Think of chemotherapy as a storm that washes away weeds in a garden; it targets rapidly dividing cancer cells.

Example: If a woman has a tumor in her breast and doctors suspect some cancer cells have spread, chemotherapy might be used to shrink the tumor before surgery or eliminate any remaining cells afterward.

Side Effects: While effective, chemotherapy can also affect healthy cells, leading to side effects like nausea, fatigue, hair loss, and an increased risk of infection.

2. Hormonal Therapy

Hormonal therapy is used for cancers that are hormone receptor-positive (HR+), meaning they grow in response to hormones like estrogen or progesterone.

How It Works: This therapy acts like a traffic cop directing hormones away from cancer cells by blocking or lowering hormone levels.

Example: For patients diagnosed with ER-positive breast cancer, medications like tamoxifen or aromatase inhibitors may be prescribed.

Side Effects: While hormonal therapy can cause hot flashes and mood changes, many patients find these effects more manageable compared to chemotherapy.

3. Targeted Therapy

Targeted therapy focuses on specific characteristics of cancer cells and is designed to attack only those cells while sparing normal ones.

How It Works: Imagine targeted therapy as a precision tool designed specifically for fixing certain problems in a machine; it hones in on particular features of cancer.

Example: For cancers that are HER2-positive (having too much of the HER2 protein), targeted treatments like trastuzumab (Herceptin) can be very effective.

Side Effects: Targeted therapies usually have different side effects than chemotherapy and may include symptoms like diarrhea and skin rashes but are generally considered less severe.

4. Immunotherapy

Immunotherapy harnesses your body's immune system to fight cancer and is becoming increasingly important in treating advanced breast cancers, particularly triple-negative breast cancer (TNBC).

How It Works: This approach boosts your immune system's ability to recognize and destroy cancer cells.

Example: Pembrolizumab (Keytruda) is an immune checkpoint inhibitor that has shown promise in treating certain cases of TNBC.

Side Effects: Side effects may include flu-like symptoms or fatigue but vary from person to person.

5. Radiation Therapy

Radiation uses high-energy waves to target specific areas where the cancer has spread (e.g., bones or brain). It can help relieve pain and improve comfort but is typically used alongside systemic therapies.

How It Works: Radiation therapy destroys cancer cells in targeted areas while minimizing damage to surrounding healthy tissue.

Example: If breast cancer has metastasized to bone causing pain, localized radiation may alleviate discomfort.
Side Effects: Side effects may include skin irritation at the treatment site and fatigue.

6. Surgery

In some cases, surgery may still be an option if tumors are causing significant pain or complications; however, this is less common in stage 4 cases.

How It Works: Surgical intervention might involve removing tumors from organs where they cause issues.

Living with Stage 4 Breast Cancer
Many individuals with stage 4 breast cancer find ways to manage their condition effectively:

- Ongoing Treatment: Regular follow-ups with healthcare teams are crucial for adjusting treatment plans based on how well the cancer responds.

- Support Systems: Emotional support from family, friends, or support groups can significantly impact coping with metastatic breast cancer.

- Palliative Care: This type of care focuses on providing relief from symptoms and improving quality of life; it can be integrated alongside other treatments or used when curative options are no longer effective.

The Importance of Communication

Open communication with healthcare providers is vital for understanding treatment options and making informed decisions about care. Don't hesitate to ask questions about your diagnosis and treatment plans; being informed helps you feel more empowered during this challenging journey.

Finding Hope

While stage 4 breast cancer presents significant challenges, advancements in treatment options offer hope for many patients. Research indicates that more women are living longer by managing the disease as a chronic illness with a focus on quality of life. Many patients find they can maintain good quality of life through ongoing treatment and support systems.

The prognosis varies significantly among individuals based on several factors including age, overall health, hormone receptor status, and specific characteristics of the tumor. Although there is no cure for stage 4 breast cancer currently available, it can often go into remission—meaning that medical professionals cannot detect it through imaging or tests.

If you or someone you love is facing stage 4 breast cancer, seeking information and support is vital. Understanding your options and maintaining open communication with your healthcare team empowers you as you navigate this journey. Each patient's experience is unique; thus, resilience and support systems play crucial roles in facing this challenge together.

With continuous advancements in research and treatment options tailored to individual needs—such as precision medicine—many patients find strength not only in their medical care but also in their ability to live meaningful lives despite their diagnosis.

Remember that while stage 4 breast cancer is serious, there remains hope through effective treatments and supportive care strategies that prioritize both longevity and quality of life.

Thinking About the Costs of Breast Cancer Surgery? Here's the Ideal Estimation Cost You Should Know

Understanding the financial implications of breast cancer surgery is crucial for patients and their families. The costs associated with breast cancer treatment can be substantial, often leading to significant financial strain. This detailed overview aims to provide insights into the costs of breast cancer surgery, factors influencing these expenses, and practical tips for managing and potentially reducing these costs.

Financial Aspects of Breast Cancer Surgery

Overview of Costs

The costs associated with breast cancer treatment vary widely depending on several factors, including the type of surgery, the stage of cancer, and the patient's insurance coverage. On average, women undergoing active treatment for breast cancer incur additional medical expenses averaging around $52,542 per person, which includes outpatient costs and prescription medications. A study indicated that women with breast cancer experience medical expenditures that are four times higher than those without the disease.

Specific surgical options also have different cost implications. For instance:

- Mastectomy (with or without reconstruction): This is often more expensive due to the complexity and length of hospital stays.

- Breast-conserving surgery (lumpectomy): Generally, less costly than mastectomy but still involves significant expenses related to follow-up treatments like radiation therapy.

Indirect Costs

In addition to direct medical expenses, patients often face indirect costs such as:
- Lost wages due to time off work for treatment.

- Travel expenses for hospital visits.

- Childcare costs during treatment periods.

Financial toxicity—a term describing the financial distress caused by medical expenses—is a significant concern for many patients. Studies show that financial burdens can lead to decreased quality of life and increased stress levels, affecting treatment adherence and overall health outcomes23.

Factors Influencing Costs

Several factors can influence the overall cost of breast cancer surgery:

- Insurance Coverage: Patients with comprehensive insurance plans may face lower out-of-pocket costs compared to those with high deductibles or limited coverage.

- Type of Surgery: As mentioned earlier, more extensive surgical options typically incur higher costs without necessarily improving outcomes3.

- Geographic Location: The cost of healthcare services varies significantly by region, affecting overall treatment expenses.

- Stage of Cancer: Advanced stages often require more aggressive (and expensive) treatments.

<u>**Tips for Managing Costs**</u>

1. **Discuss Financial Concerns with Healthcare Providers**

Patients should feel empowered to discuss financial aspects openly with their healthcare team. Research indicates that many women do not discuss costs with their doctors, despite wanting this information. Initiating these conversations can help patients understand potential expenses and explore options.

2. **Explore Financial Assistance Programs**

Many organizations offer financial assistance for cancer patients. Resources like the American Cancer Society and local charities may provide grants or help with specific costs such as transportation or medication.

3. **Consider Treatment Options Carefully**

Patients should weigh the benefits and costs of different surgical options. For example, while a double mastectomy may offer peace of mind for some, it can lead to higher costs without a significant survival benefit compared to less invasive procedures.

4. Utilize Generic Medications

Whenever possible, opt for generic versions of medications prescribed during treatment. These can significantly reduce drug costs while maintaining efficacy.

5. Investigate Payment Plans

Many hospitals offer payment plans that allow patients to spread out their medical bills over time. This can alleviate immediate financial pressure and make payments more manageable.

6. Seek Support from Nonprofits

Organizations such as Breastcancer.org provide resources on managing financial issues related to breast cancer treatment5. They often have tools to help patients navigate insurance claims and understand their benefits better.

7. Keep Detailed Records

Maintaining thorough records of all medical expenses can help in tracking spending and identifying areas where savings might be possible. This documentation is also crucial when filing claims with insurance companies or applying for aid.

Navigating the financial landscape of breast cancer surgery requires careful planning and proactive management. By understanding the potential costs involved, discussing financial concerns openly with healthcare providers, exploring assistance programs, and considering all available options, patients can mitigate some of the financial burdens associated with their treatment.

The journey through breast cancer is undoubtedly challenging, but being informed about the financial aspects can empower patients to make decisions that support both their health and financial well-being.

Effective Strategies for Utilizing the Latest Technology in Breast Cancer Detection

In today's world, technology is transforming the way we approach breast cancer detection, making it more accurate and accessible than ever before. For many women, understanding these advancements can empower them to take charge of their breast health. Here's a closer look at some of the latest technologies, their costs, and effective strategies for utilizing them in breast cancer detection.

3D Mammography (Tomosynthesis)

One of the most significant breakthroughs in breast cancer screening is 3D mammography, also known as digital breast tomosynthesis. Unlike traditional 2D mammograms that provide flat images, 3D mammography captures multiple images of the breast from different angles. This allows radiologists to examine the breast tissue layer by layer.

Why It Matters:
Research shows that 3D mammography can increase the detection rate of invasive cancers by up to 40%

compared to standard mammograms. Additionally, it reduces the number of false positives, meaning fewer women will experience the anxiety of being called back for additional tests unnecessarily.

MRI (Magnetic Resonance Imaging)

MRI is another powerful tool in breast cancer detection, especially for women at high risk or those with dense breast tissue. Unlike mammograms, MRIs use magnets and radio waves to create detailed images of the breast without exposing patients to radiation.

<u>When It's Recommended:</u>
Healthcare providers often recommend MRI as a supplemental screening tool for women with a family history of breast cancer or genetic predispositions like BRCA mutations.

Breast Ultrasound

Breast ultrasound is frequently used alongside mammography, particularly for women with dense breasts where mammograms may not be as effective. This technology uses sound waves to create images of the breast tissue and can help differentiate between solid masses and fluid-filled cysts.

Benefits:

Ultrasound is especially useful for evaluating abnormalities found on mammograms or during physical exams. It's non-invasive and does not involve radiation, making it a safe option for further investigation.

Genetic Testing and Biomarker Analysis

Advancements in genetic testing and biomarker analysis are also changing how we detect and understand breast cancer. Tests like Oncotype DX evaluate the genetic makeup of tumors to predict their behavior and response to treatment.

How This Helps:

These tests can guide treatment decisions by determining whether chemotherapy is necessary for certain patients, allowing for more personalized care.

Mobile Health Apps and Telehealth

Technology extends beyond imaging; it also encompasses how patients access care. Mobile health apps are increasingly being used to remind women about screenings and track their health data. Telehealth services allow patients to consult with specialists from home.

Understanding the Disadvantages of Advanced Breast Cancer Detection Technologies

While advancements in breast cancer detection technologies, such as 3D mammography, MRI, and genetic testing, have significantly improved early diagnosis and treatment outcomes, it's essential to consider their disadvantages as well. Understanding these limitations can help patients make informed decisions about their breast health.

Cost Considerations

One of the most significant drawbacks of advanced breast cancer detection technologies is the cost. While many of these procedures offer enhanced accuracy and benefits, they can also be expensive. For instance:

3D Mammography: Although the cost typically ranges from $100 to $300, not all insurance plans cover this advanced screening. Women without insurance or those whose plans do not include 3D mammography may face out-of-pocket expenses that can be a financial burden.

MRI: The price for a breast MRI can vary widely, often ranging from $400 to $1,500. Many patients find that their insurance may not cover MRIs unless specific criteria are met, leading to unexpected costs.

Genetic Testing: The costs for genetic tests can be staggering, ranging from $300 to $4,000. While many insurance plans cover testing for high-risk individuals, navigating the requirements for coverage can be challenging and stressful.

These financial barriers can deter women from seeking necessary screenings or following through with recommended tests, potentially delaying diagnosis and treatment.

Availability and Accessibility

Another disadvantage is the availability and accessibility of these advanced technologies. Not all healthcare facilities offer the latest imaging methods or genetic testing services. Rural areas, in particular, may lack access to specialized centers equipped with advanced diagnostic tools.

For example:

Limited Access to MRI: While MRIs are invaluable for high-risk patients or those with dense breast tissue, not every hospital or clinic has the capability to perform them. This limitation can result in longer travel times for patients seeking care, which may discourage them from pursuing necessary screenings.

Geographic Disparities: Women living in underserved communities may face significant barriers to accessing advanced technologies due to a lack of nearby facilities offering these services. This disparity can contribute to inequalities in breast cancer detection and outcomes.

Psychological Impact

The psychological impact of advanced screening technologies should not be overlooked. While these tools can provide critical information about breast health, they can also lead to increased anxiety among patients:

False Positives: Advanced technologies like 3D mammography and MRI may yield false positives—results that suggest cancer is present when it is not. This can lead to unnecessary biopsies and heightened anxiety during the waiting period for further testing.

Overdiagnosis: With improved detection capabilities comes the risk of overdiagnosis—identifying cancers that may never have caused harm during a person's lifetime. This situation can lead to overtreatment and unnecessary emotional distress for patients who might otherwise have been fine without intervention.

Need for Follow-Up Testing

Advanced technologies often lead to additional follow-up tests, which can create a cycle of anxiety and uncertainty:

Increased Testing Burden: After an initial screening reveals potential issues, patients may need further imaging or biopsies to clarify results. This process can be time-consuming and emotionally draining as patients await answers about their health.

What Makes Histopathology Essential for Diagnosing Diseases?

Histopathology plays a pivotal role in modern medicine, especially in the diagnosis and management of diseases like cancer. This field involves examining tissue samples under a microscope to identify abnormalities, including cancerous cells. Understanding how histopathology works and its significance can help demystify the diagnosis process for patients and their families.

What is Histopathology?

Histopathology is the study of tissues to diagnose diseases. In the context of breast cancer, it involves analyzing samples taken during a biopsy. These samples are prepared on slides and examined by a pathologist—a doctor who specializes in diagnosing diseases through laboratory tests. This meticulous examination provides crucial insights into the nature of the disease, guiding treatment decisions.

How Does the Process Work?

Tissue Collection: When a biopsy is performed—whether it's a fine-needle aspiration, core needle biopsy, or surgical biopsy—a small sample of breast tissue is collected.

Sample Preparation: The tissue sample is processed in a laboratory. It is fixed in formalin to preserve its structure and then embedded in paraffin wax to create thin slices for examination.

Microscopic Examination: Once prepared, the slides are stained with special dyes that highlight different cell types and structures. The pathologist examines these slides under a microscope, looking for abnormal cells that may indicate cancer.

Why Is Histopathology Important?

Histopathology provides critical information that helps guide treatment decisions. Here are some key reasons why it's essential:

Diagnosis Confirmation

Histopathology confirms whether cancer is present and helps determine the type of breast cancer (e.g., invasive ductal carcinoma or lobular carcinoma). Accurate histopathological diagnosis can lead to appropriate treatment plans tailored to specific cancer types, significantly impacting patient outcomes.

Staging and Grading

The pathologist assesses how aggressive the cancer is by examining the characteristics of the cells. This includes determining the tumor grade, which indicates how abnormal the cells look under the microscope. Higher-grade tumors tend to grow faster and may require more aggressive treatment.

Guiding Treatment Options

The results from histopathology can influence treatment decisions. For example, if the biopsy shows hormone receptor-positive breast cancer, doctors may recommend hormone therapy as part of the treatment plan.

Evidence-Based Example
A study published in the journal Cancer highlights the importance of histopathological analysis in breast cancer management. The research found that accurate histological diagnosis significantly impacts treatment outcomes, with patients receiving tailored therapies

based on their specific cancer type showing improved survival rates.

Potential Limitations

While histopathology is invaluable, there are some limitations to be aware of:

False Negatives

In rare cases, a biopsy may miss cancerous cells, leading to a false negative result. This can happen if the sampled tissue does not contain cancer or if the tumor is small and difficult to detect.

Complexity of Interpretation

Histopathological analysis requires highly trained specialists. Variability in interpretation can occur, which is why many patients seek second opinions on their pathology reports.

Histopathology is an essential component of modern medicine that plays a crucial role in diagnosing diseases like breast cancer. By providing accurate diagnoses, staging information, and guidance for treatment options, histopathologists significantly impact patient care and outcomes. Understanding this process can empower patients and their families during what can often be a challenging time.

How Does Histopathology Unlock the Power of Targeted Therapies for Cancer Treatment?

Histopathology is essential in cancer treatment as it helps doctors understand the specific characteristics of a tumor, which is crucial for selecting the right targeted therapies. When a patient is diagnosed with cancer, a sample of the tumor is taken through a biopsy. Pathologists then examine this tissue under a microscope to identify important features, such as specific proteins or genetic changes that can influence treatment options.

The Role of Histopathology in Cancer Diagnosis

One clear example is in breast cancer, where some tumors exhibit high levels of a protein called HER2. About 20-30% of breast cancers are HER2-positive, meaning they grow faster and are more aggressive.

For these patients, doctors often prescribe trastuzumab (Herceptin), a targeted therapy that specifically attacks HER2-positive cells. This targeted approach can lead to better outcomes compared to standard chemotherapy, which treats all rapidly dividing cells indiscriminately, not just the cancerous ones.

Identifying Mutations for Effective Treatment

Another critical role of histopathology is in identifying mutations that can affect treatment efficacy. For instance, in lung cancer, some patients have mutations in a gene called EGFR. Targeted therapies that inhibit EGFR can be very effective for these patients. However, over time, some tumors may develop new mutations that confer resistance to these treatments. By regularly analyzing tumor samples through histopathology, doctors can detect these changes and adjust treatment plans accordingly, switching to different therapies that may still be effective.

Advancements in Histopathological Techniques

Recent advancements in technology have also improved how we utilize histopathology in cancer treatment. Techniques like next-generation sequencing (NGS) allow doctors to analyze multiple genes simultaneously, providing a comprehensive view of the tumor's genetic landscape. This thorough analysis helps identify various potential targets for therapy, making it easier for physicians to choose the most suitable treatment options.

What Resources Are Available for Individuals with Breast Cancer Who Cannot Afford Treatment, and How Can Loved Ones Help?

Facing a breast cancer diagnosis can be an incredibly overwhelming experience, especially when financial constraints add to the stress. Fortunately, there are various resources available to assist individuals who cannot afford treatment, as well as meaningful ways that friends and family can provide support during this challenging time.

Government Assistance Programs
Medicaid

Medicaid is a state and federal program that provides health coverage for low-income individuals, including those diagnosed with breast cancer. Eligibility varies by state, but many people qualify based on income and family size. Medicaid covers a range of services, including doctor visits, hospital stays, chemotherapy, and other treatments.

How to Apply: Individuals can apply for Medicaid through their state's Medicaid office or website. It's important to check specific eligibility criteria in their state.

Medicare

Medicare is a federal health insurance program primarily for people aged 65 and older, but it also covers younger individuals with disabilities or certain medical conditions, including breast cancer. Medicare offers various plans that cover hospital care (Part A), outpatient services (Part B), and prescription drugs (Part D).

How to Apply: Eligible individuals can apply for Medicare through the Social Security Administration website or by visiting their local Social Security office. The National Breast and Cervical Cancer Early Detection Program (NBCCEDP)

This program provides access to breast cancer screening and diagnostic services for low-income, uninsured, or underinsured women. The NBCCEDP aims to detect breast cancer early when it is most treatable.

How to Access: Women can find local programs by visiting the CDC website or contacting their state health department for information about available services.

Charitable Resources

In addition to government programs, various charitable organizations offer financial assistance and support:

CancerCare: This organization provides financial assistance for treatment-related costs such as transportation, home care, and child care. They also offer counseling services and support groups.

Susan G. Komen Foundation: This foundation offers a variety of resources, including financial assistance for treatment costs and access to local support services.

BreastCancer.org Charitable Resources: This site provides a comprehensive list of charitable resources that assist individuals struggling financially with breast cancer.

How Loved Ones Can Help

If you have a friend or family member facing breast cancer without the means to afford treatment, your support can make a significant difference:

Explore Financial Assistance Together: Help them research government programs like Medicaid or Medicare and charitable organizations that may provide funds for treatment. Offer to assist in filling out applications or navigating the process.

Provide Emotional Support: Be there to listen without judgment. Encourage open communication about their feelings and fears. Suggest joining a support group where they can connect with others who understand their journey.

Assist with Practical Needs: Offer help with transportation to medical appointments or cooking meals to ensure they have nutritious food during treatment. If they have children, offer assistance with childcare or household chores.

Advocate for Their Needs: Accompany them to medical appointments to provide emotional support and help them remember important information. Research treatment options together, including clinical trials that may be available in their areas.

In summary, individuals facing breast cancer who cannot afford treatment have access to various government programs and charitable organizations that provide financial assistance. Additionally, loved ones play a crucial role in offering emotional support and practical help during this difficult time.

If you or someone you know is in need of assistance, don't hesitate to reach out to these resources or offer your support.

Remember that no one has to face this journey alone; there are people and organizations ready to help every step of the way.

What foods should be avoided when you have breast cancer?

Receiving a breast cancer diagnosis can turn your world upside down, and it often leads to a flurry of questions about treatment options, lifestyle changes, and diet. While there's no one-size-fits-all diet for breast cancer patients, certain foods may be best avoided to support overall health and well-being during treatment. Let's explore some of these foods, the reasons behind these recommendations, and also look at nutrient-rich foods that can help boost the immune system.

Foods to Avoid

Processed Foods

Processed foods often contain high levels of added sugars, unhealthy fats, and preservatives. Research has shown that diets high in processed foods can contribute to inflammation in the body, which may negatively impact cancer progression. For instance, a study published in the journal BMJ found that higher consumption of ultra-processed foods was associated with an increased risk of various cancers, including breast cancer.

Example:
Instead of potato chips or sugary cereals, opt for whole foods like fresh fruits, nuts, or yogurt.

Red and Processed Meats

High consumption of red meat (like beef and pork) and processed meats (such as bacon, sausages, and deli meats) may be linked to an increased risk of breast cancer recurrence. The World Health Organization has classified processed meats as a Group 1 carcinogen.

Example:
Swap a bacon sandwich for a hearty vegetable omelet or oatmeal topped with berries.

Sugary Drinks

Sugary beverages are loaded with added sugars that can lead to weight gain and obesity—a known risk factor for various cancers. A study published in Cancer Epidemiology Biomarkers & Prevention found that women who consumed high amounts of sugar-sweetened beverages had a greater risk of developing breast cancer.

Example:
Choose sparkling water with a splash of lemon instead of soda during lunch.

High-Fat Dairy Products
Some studies suggest that high-fat dairy products might be linked to an increased risk of breast cancer due to their saturated fat content. Opting for low-fat or plant-based alternatives may be beneficial.

Example:
Try low-fat Greek yogurt topped with fresh fruit instead of full-fat versions.

<u>Alcohol</u>
Even moderate alcohol intake can increase the risk of breast cancer recurrence. The American Cancer Society recommends limiting alcohol consumption to no more than one drink per day for women.

Example:
Alternate alcoholic drinks with water or sparkling water infused with fruit at social gatherings.

Nutrient-Rich Foods to Boost the Immune System

In addition to avoiding certain foods, incorporating nutrient-dense foods into your diet can help support your immune system during treatment:

Fruits and Vegetables:

Aim for a colorful variety like berries, leafy greens, carrots, and citrus fruits. These are rich in vitamins, antioxidants, and fiber.

Whole Grains:

Foods like quinoa, brown rice, and whole grain bread provide essential nutrients and help maintain energy levels.

Lean Proteins:
Incorporate sources like chicken, fish (especially fatty fish like salmon), beans, and legumes. Protein is crucial for healing and maintaining muscle mass.

Nuts and Seeds:

Almonds, walnuts, chia seeds, and flaxseeds are packed with healthy fats, protein, and fiber that can help reduce inflammation.

Healthy Fats:

Olive oil and avocados provide monounsaturated fats that support heart health and overall well-being.

Sample Meal Plan

Here's a simple meal plan that incorporates these nutrient-rich foods while avoiding those best left out:

Breakfast:

Overnight oats made with rolled oats topped with fresh berries and a sprinkle of chia seeds.
A cup of green tea or herbal tea.

Snack:
A small handful of almonds or walnuts.

Lunch:
Quinoa salad with mixed greens, cherry tomatoes, cucumber, chickpeas, and a dressing made from olive oil and lemon juice.
A piece of fruit (like an apple or orange).

Snack:
Low-fat Greek yogurt with sliced banana or honey.

Dinner:
Grilled salmon served with steamed broccoli and sweet potatoes.
A side salad with spinach, avocado slices, and balsamic vinaigrette.

Evening Snack (if needed):
Carrot sticks or bell pepper slices with hummus.

In summary, while navigating life after a breast cancer diagnosis can be challenging, being mindful of your diet can play a crucial role in your overall health. Avoiding processed foods, red meats, sugary drinks, high-fat dairy products, and limiting alcohol can help support your body during treatment. At the same time, incorporating nutrient-rich foods can boost your immune system and promote healing.

Always consult with your healthcare team or a registered dietitian who specializes in oncology nutrition for personalized advice tailored to your specific needs. Making informed dietary choices empowers you on your journey toward wellness and recovery.

How many years must pass for someone to be considered cancer-free?

When someone is diagnosed with breast cancer, one of the most pressing questions they often have is, "When will I be considered cancer-free?" The journey through breast cancer treatment can be long and arduous, filled with uncertainty and emotional turmoil. Understanding the timeline for being declared cancer-free can provide hope and clarity to those navigating this challenging experience.

The Five-Year Mark

In the medical community, the five-year mark is often used as a standard benchmark for determining whether a person is considered cancer-free. This doesn't mean that if you reach five years without any signs of cancer, you are guaranteed to remain cancer-free forever. Instead, it reflects a significant milestone in survival rates and the likelihood of recurrence.

Studies show that many breast cancer survivors who remain free of disease for five years after treatment have a lower risk of recurrence. According to the American Cancer Society, the five-year relative survival rate for women diagnosed with localized breast cancer is about 99%. This statistic provides a strong sense of reassurance for many patients.

Real-Life Testimonies

To illustrate this point further, let's consider some inspiring stories from well-known breast cancer survivors who have reached or surpassed that five-year mark.

Sheryl Crow

The Grammy-winning singer-songwriter Sheryl Crow was diagnosed with breast cancer in 2006. After undergoing treatment that included surgery and radiation, she has been vocal about her journey and the importance of regular screenings. Crow has shared her experience in interviews, emphasizing how reaching the five-year mark brought her immense relief and hope. She continues to advocate for breast cancer awareness and early detection, inspiring countless others with her story.

Christina Applegate

Actress Christina Applegate was diagnosed with breast cancer in 2008 at the age of 36. After opting for a double mastectomy and undergoing further treatments, she has been open about her struggles and triumphs as a survivor. In interviews, Applegate has expressed that reaching the five-year milestone gave her a renewed sense of life and purpose. She uses her platform to raise awareness about genetic testing and preventive measures for those at high risk.

Kylie Minogue

Pop icon Kylie Minogue was diagnosed with breast cancer in 2005 at the age of 36. After undergoing surgery and chemotherapy, she has spoken candidly about her journey toward recovery. In various interviews, Minogue has shared how crossing the five-year threshold felt like a significant victory. She emphasizes that while she remains vigilant about her health, reaching this milestone allowed her to embrace life more fully.

Nancy Brinker

Nancy Brinker, the founder of Susan G. Komen for the Cure, was diagnosed with breast cancer in 1980. After her treatment, she dedicated her life to raising awareness about breast cancer and advocating for research funding. Brinker's story is particularly powerful because she transformed her personal battle into a global movement that has saved countless lives. She emphasizes the importance of early detection and has been a beacon of hope for many women facing similar challenges.

Rita Wilson

Actress Rita Wilson was diagnosed with breast cancer in 2015 and underwent a double mastectomy followed by reconstructive surgery. Wilson has openly discussed her experience, including the emotional and physical challenges she faced during treatment. In interviews, she has expressed gratitude for reaching the five-year mark and emphasizes the importance of self-exams and regular check-ups. Her candidness about her journey has helped raise awareness about breast cancer and the importance of support systems during treatment.

Giuliana Rancic

Television personality Giuliana Rancic was diagnosed with breast cancer in 2011 at the age of 36. After undergoing a double mastectomy and subsequent treatments, she has become an advocate for breast cancer awareness. Rancic often shares her story on social media and in interviews, highlighting the emotional aspects of her journey and how reaching significant milestones, like being cancer-free for several years, has impacted her outlook on life.

Hoda Kotb

Hoda Kotb, co-anchor of the "Today" show, is another inspiring figure. While she is not a breast cancer survivor herself, she has been a powerful advocate for awareness and early detection after losing her mother to breast cancer. Kotb often shares stories of survivors on her show, emphasizing the importance of community support and resilience in the face of adversity.

Beyond Five Years

While the five-year mark is significant, it's important to remember that every individual's journey is unique. Some survivors may experience recurrence after five years, while others may continue to thrive long after that point without any issues. Many healthcare providers now emphasize long-term follow-up care rather than simply focusing on a specific timeline.

Breast cancer survivors often report that their experiences shape their perspectives on life. They learn to celebrate small victories and cherish each day. For many, being "cancer-free" becomes not just about medical definitions but also about living fully and embracing life after treatment. And physically exhausting. Knowing more about the chances of recurrence can help patients and their loved ones navigate the path ahead with greater awareness and preparedness.

Is There a Possibility That Breast Cancer Will Return After Treatment Has Been Completed?

After completing treatment for breast cancer, many survivors are filled with hope and relief. However, it's natural to wonder about the possibility of recurrence—whether the cancer could return. Understanding the factors that influence recurrence and knowing what steps to take if it happens can empower individuals on their journey to recovery.

Understanding Recurrence

Breast cancer recurrence refers to the return of cancer after treatment, which can happen in several ways:

- Local Recurrence: This occurs when cancer returns to the same breast or chest area where it was originally diagnosed.

- Regional Recurrence: This type happens when cancer returns to nearby lymph nodes.

- Distant Recurrence (Metastasis): This occurs when cancer spreads to other parts of the body, such as bones, liver, lungs, or brain.

The risk of recurrence varies based on several factors, including:
Stage of Cancer at Diagnosis: More advanced stages often carry a higher risk of recurrence.

Type of Breast Cancer: Certain types, like triple-negative breast cancer, may have a higher likelihood of returning.

- Response to Treatment: How the cancer responded to initial treatments can also impact recurrence rates.

- Hormone Receptor Status: Hormone receptor-positive cancers may have different patterns of recurrence compared to hormone receptor-negative cancers.

Studies show that breast cancer can recur at any time after treatment, but most recurrences happen within the first five years. However, some patients may experience recurrences even after ten years or more.

What to Do If Breast Cancer Returns

If breast cancer does return, it's important not to panic. Here are steps and recommendations for navigating this challenging situation:

Consult Your Healthcare Team: The first step is to reach out to your oncologist or healthcare provider. They will conduct tests to determine the location and extent of the recurrence and develop a new treatment plan tailored to your situation.

Consider Treatment Options:

- Surgery: Depending on where the cancer has returned, surgery may be an option. This could involve a lumpectomy or mastectomy.

- Radiation Therapy: If the recurrence is localized, radiation therapy might be recommended.

- Systemic Treatments: These could include chemotherapy, hormonal therapy, or targeted therapy based on the characteristics of the cancer.

- Clinical Trials: Ask about clinical trials that may offer access to new therapies or approaches that are not yet widely available.

- Emotional Support: A recurrence can be emotionally taxing. Consider seeking support from friends, family, or professional counselors. Joining a support group for breast cancer survivors can also provide comfort and understanding from those who have faced similar challenges.

- Lifestyle Changes: Focus on maintaining a healthy lifestyle through balanced nutrition, regular exercise, and stress management techniques. Some studies suggest that lifestyle factors can play a role in reducing the risk of recurrence.

- Regular Follow-Ups: After treatment for a recurrence, regular follow-up appointments are crucial for monitoring health and addressing any concerns early on.

While there is a possibility that breast cancer may return after treatment has been completed, understanding this risk can help individuals prepare for their journey ahead. If recurrence occurs, it's essential to consult with healthcare professionals who can guide you through the next steps and create a personalized treatment plan.

Is There Evidence Linking Underwire Bras or Antiperspirants to Increased Breast Cancer Risk?

Concerns about breast cancer risk often led to questions about everyday items like underwire bras and personal care products such as antiperspirants and deodorants. Many women wonder if these items could contribute to their risk of developing breast cancer. However, current scientific evidence does not support these claims.

Underwire Bras

The debate over whether wearing underwire bras increases breast cancer risk has circulated for years. However, research indicates that there is no causal link between wearing underwire bras and an increased risk of breast cancer. The American Cancer Society states that there is no evidence to suggest that bras, underwire or otherwise, cause breast cancer. Additionally, a study published in the Journal of the National Cancer Institute found no association between bra style and breast cancer risk.

The confusion surrounding this topic may stem from misconceptions about how breast cancer develops. Factors such as genetics, hormonal levels, and lifestyle choices play a more significant role in breast cancer risk than the type of bra a woman chooses to wear.

Antiperspirants and Deodorants

Similarly, concerns about antiperspirants and deodorants contributing to breast cancer risk have been addressed by multiple studies. A comprehensive review published in the Journal of the National Cancer Institute found no evidence linking the use of these products to an increased risk of breast cancer. The American Cancer Society also affirms that there is no conclusive evidence supporting this claim.

One primary concern has been the aluminum compounds found in antiperspirants, which temporarily block sweat glands. Some theories suggested that these compounds could be absorbed through the skin and disrupt hormonal balance, potentially leading to breast cancer. However, research has shown that the amount of aluminum absorbed through the skin is minimal and not sufficient to pose a health risk. Additionally, a study published in Cancer Causes & Control concluded that there was no significant association between antiperspirant use and breast cancer risk, further reinforcing the idea that these products are safe for everyday use.

Both underwire bras and antiperspirants have been scrutinized for their potential links to breast cancer; however, current evidence from reputable studies and health organizations indicates that there is no credible connection between these items and an increased risk of developing breast cancer. Women can feel confident in their choices regarding undergarments and personal care products without fear of contributing to their cancer risk.

Can Soursop, Mangosteen, and Green Tea Unlock the Secrets to Beating Breast Cancer?

In recent years, many natural remedies have gained popularity as potential treatments for various health conditions, including cancer. Among these are soursop (also known as graviola), mangosteen, and green tea. Some proponents claim that these foods possess extraordinary healing properties, suggesting that they may be more effective than conventional treatments like chemotherapy. However, it is essential to examine these claims critically and understand what the scientific community has to say.

Soursop: The Fruit of Controversy

Soursop has been touted for its potential anti-cancer properties due to its high content of antioxidants and phytochemicals. A study published in the Journal of Natural Products highlighted those compounds extracted from soursop exhibited cytotoxic effects on various cancer cell lines, including breast cancer cells (Feng et al., 2015). However, while laboratory studies show promise, it is crucial to note that these results do not translate directly into clinical efficacy in humans.

The American Cancer Society emphasizes that while some laboratory studies suggest potential benefits, there is no substantial evidence from clinical trials that soursop can cure cancer or replace conventional treatments. Additionally, consuming soursop in large quantities may pose risks due to its neurotoxic properties, which have been linked to movement disorders similar to Parkinson's disease (Pérez et al., 2017).

Mangosteen: The Queen of Fruits

Mangosteen is another fruit that has garnered attention for its purported health benefits. Rich in xanthones—antioxidant compounds—mangosteen has been studied for its anti-inflammatory and anti-cancer properties. A review published in Phytotherapy Research noted that xanthones could inhibit cancer cell proliferation and induce apoptosis (programmed cell death) in various cancer types (Shah et al., 2016).

However, while these findings are promising, they primarily derive from laboratory studies rather than human trials. The National Cancer Institute states that there is currently insufficient evidence to support the use of mangosteen as a treatment for cancer. As with soursop, more research is needed to determine its effectiveness and safety in humans.

Green Tea: A More Established Ally

Green tea has long been celebrated for its health benefits, particularly due to its high levels of catechins—powerful antioxidants. Several studies have suggested that green tea consumption may be associated with a reduced risk of developing certain types of cancer, including breast cancer. A meta-analysis published in Breast Cancer Research and Treatment found that women who consumed green tea regularly had a lower risk of breast cancer recurrence compared to those who did not (Zhang et al., 2019).

While green tea shows promise as a complementary approach to cancer prevention and management due to its antioxidant properties, it is essential to clarify that it is not a cure for breast cancer. The American Institute for Cancer Research recommends incorporating green tea into a balanced diet but emphasizes that it should not replace conventional treatment methods.

A Cautious Approach

While soursop, mangosteen, and green tea offer intriguing possibilities as part of a healthy diet, it is crucial to approach claims regarding their effectiveness against breast cancer with caution. Current scientific evidence does not support the idea that these foods can cure breast cancer or serve as substitutes for established treatments like chemotherapy.

For anyone facing a breast cancer diagnosis or seeking information about treatment options, consulting healthcare professionals is vital. They can provide guidance based on the latest research and help patients make informed decisions about their care.

In summary, while incorporating fruits like soursop and mangosteen and beverages like green tea into your diet can contribute to overall health and wellness, it's essential to rely on evidence-based treatments when addressing serious conditions like breast cancer.

Can Hormonal Therapy Cause Ovarian Thickening? Understanding Tamoxifen's Effects

When it comes to breast cancer treatment, hormonal therapy plays a crucial role, particularly for patients with hormone receptor-positive tumors. Among the various medications used, tamoxifen is one of the most commonly prescribed. While tamoxifen has been shown to be effective in reducing the risk of cancer recurrence, many patients wonder about its side effects, including whether it can cause changes in ovarian health, such as thickening of the ovarian lining.

What Is Tamoxifen and How Does It Work?

Tamoxifen is a selective estrogen receptor modulator (SERM) that blocks estrogen receptors in breast tissue. This action helps prevent estrogen from fueling the growth of certain types of breast cancer. According to the American Society of Clinical Oncology (ASCO), tamoxifen is often prescribed for five to ten years after initial treatment to lower the risk of recurrence and improve survival rates.

Can Tamoxifen Cause Ovarian Thickening?

Yes, tamoxifen can potentially lead to changes in the ovaries, including thickening of the ovarian lining (endometrial hyperplasia). This occurs because tamoxifen has estrogen-like effects on certain tissues, particularly the endometrium (the lining of the uterus). While it blocks estrogen in breast tissue, it can stimulate estrogen receptors in other areas, such as the uterus and ovaries.

Research Insights

A study published in The Journal of Clinical Oncology found that women taking tamoxifen had a higher incidence of endometrial changes compared to those not on hormonal therapy. The study indicated that approximately 20% of women on tamoxifen experienced some degree of endometrial thickening (Parker et al., 2019).

Common Effects of Tamoxifen on the Body

While tamoxifen can be beneficial in managing breast cancer, it also comes with a range of potential side effects that patients should be aware of:

1. **Menstrual Changes:**

Many women report alterations in their menstrual cycles while on tamoxifen. This can include irregular periods or changes in flow.

2. **Hot Flashes:**

Hot flashes are one of the most common side effects associated with tamoxifen. According to a study by the National Cancer Institute, nearly 60-70% of women experience hot flashes while undergoing treatment.

3. **Weight Gain:**

Some patients may experience weight gain during treatment. A review published in Breast Cancer Research and Treatment noted that hormonal therapies could contribute to metabolic changes leading to weight fluctuations (Bae et al., 2020).

4. **Mood Swings:**

Hormonal fluctuations caused by tamoxifen can also affect mood. Some women report increased anxiety or depressive symptoms during treatment.

5. Increased Risk of Endometrial Cancer:

While rare, there is an increased risk of endometrial cancer associated with long-term use of tamoxifen due to its stimulating effect on the uterine lining. Women are advised to have regular gynecological check-ups while on this medication.

What Body Parts Should Be Monitored After Breast Cancer Treatment?

After undergoing breast cancer treatment, it is crucial to remain vigilant about monitoring various aspects of your health, as the aftermath can bring about significant changes in your body. In the United States, approximately 1 in 8 women will be diagnosed with breast cancer in their lifetime, with an estimated 310,720 new cases expected in 2024 alone. This statistic underscores the importance of awareness and proactive health management after treatment. One of the primary areas to keep an eye on is your breasts.

After surgery, you may notice alterations in size, shape, or texture, and it's essential to be aware of any swelling or pain in the treated area. Surgical procedures like mastectomy or lumpectomy can lead to noticeable changes that might affect not only how your breasts look but also how you feel about yourself. Regular self-exams and follow-up appointments with your healthcare provider become vital tools for catching any unusual changes early, helping you address potential issues before they escalate.

Another important area to monitor is your ovaries. Many women experience irregular menstrual cycles or missed periods following treatment, along with symptoms of menopause such as hot flashes or night sweats. Chemotherapy and certain hormonal therapies can impact ovarian function, potentially leading to early menopause or fertility challenges.

By keeping track of these changes, you can gain insights into how your body is responding to treatment and discuss any concerns with your doctor. It's worth noting that the emotional and physical toll of these changes can be significant; therefore, open communication with healthcare providers about menstrual health is essential.

It's also crucial to pay attention to your lymph nodes. If lymph nodes were removed during surgery or affected by radiation, you might notice swelling or discomfort in the armpit or neck area. Additionally, some patients develop lymphedema, characterized by swelling due to fluid buildup. Monitoring these symptoms closely allows for early intervention and management strategies that can significantly improve your quality of life.

Studies indicate that up to 20% to 30% of patients who undergo axillary lymph node dissection may experience lymphedema at some point after treatment.

Your skin is another area that requires attention. Radiation therapy can lead to changes in skin texture and color, causing sensitivity or irritation in the treated area. It's important to watch for persistent redness or rashes and address any skin issues promptly with appropriate skincare products recommended by your healthcare team. Research has shown that maintaining good skin care practices post-treatment can help mitigate some side effects associated with radiation.

Moreover, don't overlook your heart health. Treatments for breast cancer—particularly certain chemotherapy regimens and radiation targeting the chest area—can have implications for cardiovascular health. Be alert for signs such as unexplained fatigue, shortness of breath, chest pain, or swelling in the legs and feet. Regular check-ups that include heart function assessments are essential for identifying potential issues early on; studies have indicated that certain chemotherapy drugs may increase the risk of heart problems later in life.

Additionally, keep an eye on your bone health. Hormonal therapies used in breast cancer treatment can weaken bones over time, increasing the risk of osteoporosis. Be aware of any increased bone pain or fractures and discuss these concerns with your doctor. Engaging in weight-bearing exercises and ensuring adequate intake of calcium and vitamin D can help support bone strength; it's estimated that women undergoing aromatase inhibitor therapy may lose up to 1% to 2% of bone density each year.

Lastly, mental health cannot be overlooked during this recovery phase. The emotional toll of a cancer diagnosis and its treatment can manifest as anxiety, depression, mood swings, or difficulty concentrating. It's essential to monitor your emotional well-being and seek support when needed—whether through counseling services, support groups, or open conversations with loved ones.

Research indicates that up to 40% of cancer survivors experience psychological distress post-treatment; thus, addressing mental health is just as critical as monitoring physical health.

By remaining proactive about these key areas—your breasts, ovaries, lymph nodes, skin, heart health, bone health, and mental well-being—you empower yourself to take charge of your recovery journey after breast cancer treatment. This vigilance not only enhances your quality of life but also ensures that any concerns are addressed promptly and effectively. With over 4 million breast cancer survivors currently living in the United States—a testament to advances in early detection and treatment—staying informed and engaged in your health care can lead to better outcomes and a fulfilling life beyond cancer.

Your Guide to Pregnancy After Breast Cancer: Empowering Choices for the Future

Facing a breast cancer diagnosis is a life-altering experience, and for many women, the desire to start or grow a family remains a priority. If you're navigating life after breast cancer and considering pregnancy, it's essential to understand the implications, timelines, and options available to you. This article will equip you with the knowledge and steps necessary to make informed decisions about pregnancy post-cancer.

Understanding the Risks: Why Timing Matters

Action Step: Consult Your Healthcare Team
Before making any decisions about pregnancy, schedule a consultation with your oncologist and a fertility specialist. They can provide personalized advice based on your treatment history and current health status.

Recommended Waiting Period

Most doctors advise waiting at least two years after completing treatment before trying to conceive. This period allows your body to recover fully and reduces the risk of recurrence during a critical time.

Why Wait?

- Recurrence Risk: The likelihood of breast cancer returning is highest in the first two years post-treatment. Waiting helps ensure that you are in a stable health position before embarking on pregnancy.

- Health Monitoring: This waiting period allows for regular follow-ups with your healthcare team to monitor your health and manage any potential complications.

Contraceptive Options During Treatment

Action Step: Choose the Right Contraception
If you are undergoing treatment, it's crucial to avoid pregnancy. Discuss contraceptive options with your healthcare provider to find the best fit for your situation.

Effective Methods:

- Barrier Methods: Use condoms or cervical caps, which do not interfere with hormonal treatments.

- IUDs: Consider a hormone-free intrauterine device (IUD) for long-term contraception without hormonal side effects.

- Emergency Contraception: If needed, emergency contraceptive pills are generally safe for breast cancer survivors.

Methods to Avoid

Hormonal Contraceptives: Steer clear of hormonal methods like the combined contraceptive pill or hormonal IUDs due to potential risks associated with hormone-sensitive breast cancers.

Exploring Fertility Options

Action Step: Assess Your Fertility Status

If you're concerned about your fertility after treatment, take proactive steps to evaluate your options:

- Fertility Assessment: Speak with a fertility specialist about fertility preservation methods available before starting treatment. Techniques such as egg freezing can provide future options for conception.

- Understand Your Chances: Many women can conceive naturally after treatment, but some may face challenges. A fertility assessment can help clarify your situation.

Preparing for Pregnancy

Action Step: Create a Comprehensive Plan
Once you've consulted with your healthcare team and decided to pursue pregnancy, develop a detailed plan:

1. **Health Optimization:**

Focus on maintaining a healthy lifestyle through balanced nutrition, regular exercise, and stress management techniques.

Schedule regular check-ups with both your oncologist and obstetrician to ensure ongoing health monitoring.

2. Emotional Support:

Pregnancy after cancer can be emotionally complex. Seek support from counselors or support groups specializing in cancer survivorship and pregnancy.

Engage with others who have had similar experiences through online forums or local support networks.

3. Educate Yourself:

Read books and resources about pregnancy after cancer. Knowledge will empower you throughout this journey.

Understanding Pregnancy Risks

While studies indicate that pregnancy does not increase the risk of breast cancer recurrence for most women, it's essential to discuss any specific concerns with your healthcare provider. They can help you weigh the benefits and risks based on your unique circumstances.

Taking Action During Pregnancy

Action Step: Stay Engaged with Your Healthcare Team
Once pregnant, maintain open lines of communication
with both your obstetrician and oncologist:

Regular Check-Ups: Schedule frequent
appointments to monitor both your health and that of
your baby.

Discuss Any Concerns: Be proactive in discussing
any changes in your health or emotional well-being
during pregnancy.

Pregnancy after breast cancer is not only possible but
can also be a fulfilling part of your life journey. By
taking informed actions—consulting healthcare
professionals, understanding fertility options, and
creating a supportive environment—you empower
yourself to navigate this path confidently.

Is Pain After Surgery and Tumor Removal a Side Effect? Understanding the Causes

Experiencing pain after surgery, particularly following a procedure like tumor removal, is a common concern for many patients. This discomfort can be attributed to several factors, and understanding these can help alleviate worries about what you're feeling.

1. Post-Surgical Pain

What It Is: After any surgical procedure, including tumor removal, it's normal to experience some level of pain. This is often due to the body's natural healing process. The surgical site may be sore as tissues heal, and this pain can vary in intensity from mild discomfort to more significant pain.

Why It Happens:

During surgery, incisions are made, and tissues are manipulated or removed. This can lead to inflammation and irritation in the surrounding areas, which triggers pain signals. According to the American Society of Clinical Oncology, post-operative pain is a common experience and usually improves over time as healing progresses.

2. Nerve Sensitivity

What It Is: Sometimes, nerves in the area where surgery was performed can become sensitive or irritated. This can lead to sensations of sharp pain, tingling, or numbness.

Why It Happens:

Surgical procedures can sometimes affect nearby nerves. As these nerves heal, they may send mixed signals to the brain, resulting in discomfort. This phenomenon is known as neuropathic pain and can occur after various types of surgery.

3. Impact of Weather

What It Is: Some individuals report increased pain during cold weather or changes in humidity. This is often described as "weather-related pain."

Why It Happens:

Cold temperatures can cause muscles and joints to tighten, which may exacerbate existing pain from surgical sites. Additionally, changes in atmospheric pressure can affect how our bodies feel pain. While this is not directly related to the surgery itself, it can influence how you perceive discomfort.

4. **Psychological Factors**

What It Is: Emotional well-being plays a significant role in how we experience pain. Anxiety or stress about recovery can amplify feelings of discomfort.

Why It Happens:
The mind and body are closely connected; stress hormones can heighten sensitivity to pain. Post-surgical anxiety is common and can make it feel like recovery is more painful than it actually is.

Remember, experiencing pain after surgery and tumor removal is typically a normal part of the healing process. While weather changes may influence your perception of this pain, it's essential to recognize that post-surgical discomfort often stems from the body's natural response to surgery and healing.

If you find that your pain is severe or worsening over time, or if you have concerns about your recovery, it's important to consult with your healthcare provider.

They can assess your condition and provide appropriate guidance or treatment options to help manage your symptoms effectively.

Embracing Your Journey

As you close this eBook, take a moment to breathe and reflect on what you've learned. The journey through breast health and cancer awareness is deeply personal and often filled with a mix of emotions—fear, hope, uncertainty, and strength. You've taken a significant step by seeking knowledge, and that alone is an act of courage.

Throughout these pages, we've explored important questions and shared insights that empower you to take charge of your health. Remember, knowledge is not just power; it's a bridge that connects you to your healthcare team and your own inner strength. By understanding your body and the changes it undergoes, you become your own best advocate.

Finding Hope in Every Step

It's completely normal to feel a whirlwind of emotions as you navigate this path. Allow yourself to feel whatever comes up—those feelings are valid and part of your unique story. Lean on your support system—friends, family, or support groups—those who understand what you're going through. They can provide comfort when the road feels rocky.

As you look ahead, embrace the possibilities that each new day brings. Whether it's finding joy in small moments or pursuing passions that light up your spirit, prioritize what makes you feel alive. Healing is not just about the physical; it's about nurturing your heart and mind too.

Your Story Matters Your journey is powerful. Sharing your experiences can inspire others who may be facing similar challenges. Your voice carries weight—don't hesitate to use it. Every question you ask and every step you take is a testament to your resilience.

In closing, may you continue to seek knowledge, nurture yourself, and embrace the journey ahead with an open heart. You are not alone; there's a community ready to support you as you navigate this path toward health and wellness.

Thank you for letting us be part of your journey. Here's to new beginnings, renewed hope, and the incredible strength that lies within you.

--- END ---

References

American Cancer Society. (n.d.). "Breast Cancer." Retrieved from American Cancer Society.

American Cancer Society. (n.d.). "Bras and Breast Cancer Risk." Retrieved from American Cancer Society.

American Cancer Society. (n.d.). "Antiperspirants and Breast Cancer." Retrieved from American Cancer Society.

Colditz, G.A., & Rosner, B.A. (2000). "Risk Factors for Breast Cancer." Journal of the National Cancer Institute, 92(13), 1050-1061. DOI: 10.1093/jnci/92.13.1050.

McGrath, C., et al. (2003). "Antiperspirant Use and Breast Cancer Risk." Cancer Causes & Control, 14(8), 741-746. DOI: 10.1023/A:1026110802115.

MyBCTeam. (n.d.). "Which Types of Breast Cancer Have the Highest Recurrence Rate?" Retrieved from MyBCTeam.

U.S. Preventive Services Task Force (USPSTF). (2016). "Screening for Breast Cancer: U.S. Preventive Services Task Force Recommendation Statement." JAMA, 315(16), 1738-1747. DOI: 10.1001/jama.2016.2901.

National Comprehensive Cancer Network (NCCN). (2023). "NCCN Clinical Practice Guidelines in Oncology: Breast Cancer." Retrieved from NCCN.
World Health Organization (WHO). (2021). "Breast cancer." Retrieved from WHO.

Breastcancer.org. (n.d.). "Breast Cancer Risk Factors." Retrieved from Breastcancer.org.

National Cancer Institute (NCI). (2021). "Breast Cancer Treatment (PDQ®)–Patient Version." Retrieved from NCI.

Centers for Disease Control and Prevention (CDC). (2022). "Breast Cancer Statistics." Retrieved from CDC.

American Society of Clinical Oncology (ASCO). (2021). "Breast Cancer: Overview." Retrieved from ASCO.

Komen, S.G. Foundation. (n.d.). "What is Breast Cancer?" Retrieved from Susan G. Komen Foundation.

The Lancet Oncology. (2018). "Global Burden of Breast Cancer." The Lancet Oncology, 19(2), e92-e93. DOI: 10.1016/S1470-2045(18)30050-5.

Feng, R., et al. (2015). "Cytotoxicity of Graviola Extracts on Human Breast Cancer Cells." Journal of Natural Products.

Pérez, J., et al. (2017). "Neurotoxicity Associated with Graviola Consumption." Toxicology Reports.

Shah, S.A., et al. (2016). "Anticancer Potential of Xanthones from Mangosteen: A Review." Phytotherapy Research.
Zhang, Y., et al. (2019). "Green Tea Consumption and Breast Cancer Risk: A Meta-Analysis." Breast Cancer Research and Treatment.